Over 32,000 Baby Names

Baby Names from A to Z

Veronica Utley

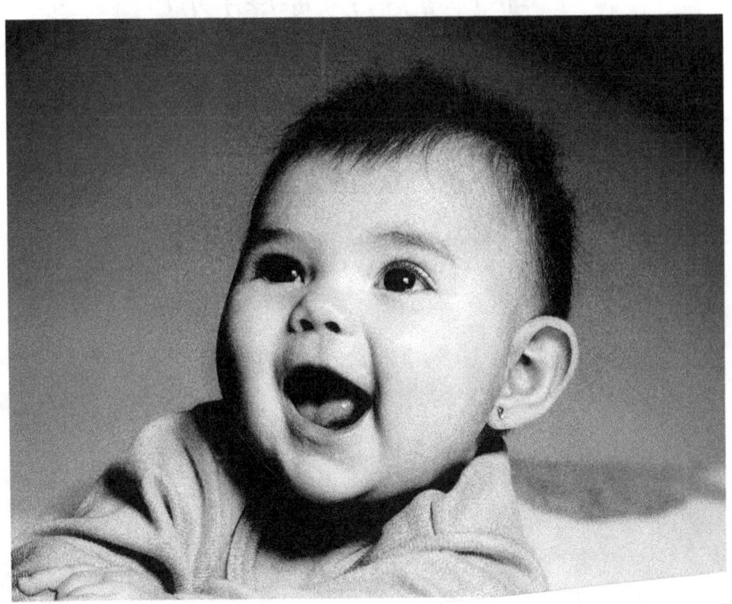

Cover and page design by Veronica Utley

Printed by CreateSpace

First edition published 2017

ISBN-13: 978-1978338999

ISBN-10: 1978338996

Introduction

As a mother myself, I know that every child is unique. This is why, upon trying to find a name for my two beautiful daughters, I eschewed the traditional and the conformist, and decided to pick a name that wasn't bound by the oppresive rules of tradition.

I made sure to give them names that matched their personalities exactly in the way they sounded.

However, I did not have the advantage of a good, comprehensive book of names to choose from - instead, I put in a lot of painstaking work and research in finding names for my daughters.

In any case, I am proud to call Shazeda and Nneka my daughters. Both of them are now old enough to both appreciate their names aren't common names (especially living here in the UK), but also old enough to enjoy their unique names.

I have asked them a few times that - if they had the opportunity - would they change their names? Neither of them could even dream of parting with their names.

This book provides one of the most comprehensive lists of modern baby names, and I hope that this compilation of names will help you choose a name for your child that you feel is right for them.

- Veronica

A

A	AAHAAN	AALIYAH-ROSE
A-JAY	AAHAD	AALIYAN
A.J.	AAHAN	AALIYHA
A'ISHA	AAHANA	AALLIYAH
A'ISHAH	AAHIL	AALYA
A'NIYAH	AAHNA	AALYAH
AA'ISHA	AAIDAH	AALYIAH
AA'ISHAH	AAILA	AAMAAL
AABAN	AAILYAH	AAMAL
AABID	AAIMA	AAMAN
AABIDAH	AAINA	AAMANAH
AABISH	AAIRA	AAMANEE
AADAM	AAIRAH	AAMANI
AADAN	AAISHA	AAMAR
AADARSH	AAISHAH	AAMAYA
AADEN	AAIZA	AAMENA
AADESH	AAIZAH	AAMENAH
AADHAM	AAJAY	AAMER
AADHAV	AAKARSH	AAMIL
AADHEEN	AAKASH	AAMILAH
AADHI	AAKIF	AAMINA
AADHIRA	AAKIFA	AAMINAH
AADHITHYA	AAKIFAH	AAMIR
AADHVIK	AAKRITI	AAMIRA
AADHYA	AALA	AAMIRAH
AADI	AALAA	AAMIYAH
AADIDEV	AALAYA	AAMNA
AADIL	AALAYAH	AAMNAH
AADILA	AALEAH	AANA
AADILAH	AALEEN	AANAV
AADIT	AALEIGHA	AANAY
AADITRI	AALEYAH	AANAYA
AADITYA	AALIA	AANCHAL
AADVIK	AALIAH	AANIA
AADYA	AALIM	AANIKA
AAEESHA	AALIMAH	AANIS
AAFIA	AALISHA	AANISAH
AAFIYA	AALIYA	AANISHA
AAFIYAH	AALIYAAN	AANIYA
AAFREEN	AALIYAH	AANIYAH
AAFRIN	AALIYAH-GRACE	AANVI
	AALIYAH-JADE	AANYA
	AALIYAH-LOUISE	AAQIB
	AALIYAH-MAE	AAQIL
	AALIYAH-MAI	AARA
	AALIYAH-MARIE	AARABI
	AALIYAH-MAY	AARADHYA
	AALIYAH-RAE	AARAF

AARAIZ	AARTI	AATIQA
AARALYN	AARUHI	AATIQAH
AARAN	AARUN	AATISH
AARANI	AARUSAN	AAVA
AARATHANA	AARUSH	AAVAI
AARAV	AARUSHI	AAVISH
AAREN	AARVI	AAVNI
AAREZ	AARVIN	AAVYA
AARI	AARY	AAYA
AARIA	AARYA	AAYAAN
AARIAH	AARYAHI	AAYAH
AARIAN	AARYAN	AAYAN
AARIANA	AARYANA	AAYANA
AARIB	AARYANNA	AAYANSH
AARIC	AARYAV	AAYAT
AARIF	AARYN	AAYATH
AARIFA	AARYUN	AAYDEN
AARIFAH	AARYZ	AAYESHA
AARIKA	AARZO	AAYLA
AARIN	AARZOO	AAYLIAH
AARINI	AARZU	AAYMA
AARIS	AASHA	AAYRA
AARISH	AASHI	AAYRAH
AARISHA	AASHIKA	AAYSHA
AARIT	AASHIR	AAYUSH
AARIV	AASHISH	AAYUSHI
AARIYA	AASHIYANA	AAYZA
AARIYAH	AASHMAN	AAZAN
AARIYAN	AASHNA	AAZEEN
AARIZ	AASHNI	AAZIL
AARNA	AASHRITHA	ABA
AARNAV	AASHRIYA	ABAAN
AARO	AASHVI	ABAAS
AAROHI	AASIA	ABAGAEL
AARON	AASIF	ABAGAIL
AARON-JAMES	AASIM	ABAIGEAL
AARON-JAY	AASIYA	ABAN
AARON-JOHN	AASIYAH	ABANOUB
AARON-JUNIOR	AASTHA	ABAS
AARON-LEE	AATHAVAN	ABASS
AARONAS	AATHAVI	ABAYOMI
AARONDEEP	AATHIRA	ABBA
AARONJIT	AATHIRAN	ABBAAS
AARONVEER	AATHISH	ABBAS
AAROON	AATIF	ABBASS
AARRON	AATIFA	ABBE
AARSH	AATIKA	ABBEE
AARTHI	AATIKAH	ABBEY

ABBEY-LEIGH	ABDELAZIZ	ABDIWAHID
ABBEY-LOUISE	ABDELKADER	ABDIWALI
ABBEYGAIL	ABDELKARIM	ABDOU
ABBEYGALE	ABDELLAH	ABDOUL
ABBEYGAYLE	ABDELMALEK	ABDOULAYE
ABBI	ABDELMOUMEN	ABDOULIE
ABBI-LEIGH	ABDELRAHIM	ABDOULLAH
ABBI-LOUISE	ABDELRAHMAN	ABDOURAHMAN
ABBI-MAE	ABDELRAHMANE	ABDRAHMAN
ABBIE	ABDERAHMAN	ABDU
ABBIE-GAIL	ABDERAHMANE	ABDUALLAH
ABBIE-GAYLE	ABDERRAHMAN	ABDUL
ABBIE-GRACE	ABDERRAHMANE	ABDUL-
ABBIE-JAI	ABDI	ABDUL-AHAD
ABBIE-JANE	ABDIASIS	ABDUL-ALEEM
ABBIE-JO	ABDIAZIZ	ABDUL-AZEEZ
ABBIE-LEA	ABDIFATAH	ABDUL-AZIZ
ABBIE-LEE	ABDIHAFID	ABDUL-BAASIT
ABBIE-LEIGH	ABDIHAKIM	ABDUL-BASIT
ABBIE-LOUISE	ABDIHAKIN	ABDUL-HAADI
ABBIE-MAE	ABDIHAMID	ABDUL-HADI
ABBIE-MAI	ABDIKADIR	ABDUL-HAKEEM
ABBIE-MAY	ABDIKARIM	ABDUL-HAKIM
ABBIE-ROSE	ABDIKARIN	ABDUL-HANNAN
ABBIEGAIL	ABDIKHALIQ	ABDUL-HASEEB
ABBIEGALE	ABDILADIF	ABDUL-KAREEM
ABBIEGAYLE	ABDILAHI	ABDUL-KARIM
ABBIELEIGH	ABDILLAHI	ABDUL-LATEEF
ABBIELOUISE	ABDIMAJID	ABDUL-MALIK
ABBIGAIL	ABDIMAJIID	ABDUL-MANNAN
ABBIGALE	ABDIMALIK	ABDUL-MATEEN
ABBIGAYLE	ABDINASIR	ABDUL-MOMIN
ABBY	ABDINUR	ABDUL-MUIZ
ABBY-LEIGH	ABDIQANI	ABDUL-NASIR
ABBY-MAY	ABDIRAHIIM	ABDUL-QADIR
ABBY-ROSE	ABDIRAHIM	ABDUL-QAYYUM
ABBYGAEL	ABDIRAHMAAN	ABDUL-RAHEEM
ABBYGAIL	ABDIRAHMAN	ABDUL-RAHIM
ABBYGALE	ABDIRASHID	ABDUL-RAHMAN
ABBYGAYLE	ABDIRAXMAN	ABDUL-REHMAN
ABD	ABDIRAZAQ	ABDUL-SAMAD
ABDAAL	ABDIRISAK	ABDUL-SAMI
ABDAL	ABDIRISAQ	ABDUL-WADOOD
ABDALLA	ABDIRIZAK	ABDUL-WAHAAB
ABDALLAH	ABDISALAM	ABDUL-WAHAB
ABDALRAHMAN	ABDISAMAD	ABDUL-WAHHAB
ABDARAHMAN	ABDISHAKUR	ABDUL-WASAY
ABDEL	ABDIWAHAB	ABDULA

ABDULAAHI	ABDUR	ABHINAV
ABDULAH	ABDUR-RAFAY	ABHIRAJ
ABDULAHAD	ABDUR-RAHEEM	ABHIRAM
ABDULAHI	ABDUR-RAHIM	ABHIRAMI
ABDULAI	ABDUR-RAHMAAN	ABHISHEK
ABDULALEEM	ABDUR-RAHMAN	ABI
ABDULAZEEZ	ABDUR-REHMAN	ABI-LEIGH
ABDULAZIZ	ABDURAHEEM	ABI-LOUISE
ABDULBASIT	ABDURAHIM	ABI-MAE
ABDULFATAH	ABDURAHMAN	ABI-ROSE
ABDULHAADI	ABDURRAHEEM	ABIA
ABDULHADI	ABDURRAHIM	ABIBAT
ABDULHAKEEM	ABDURRAHMAAN	ABIBATU
ABDULHAKIM	ABDURRAHMAN	ABID
ABDULHALIM	ABDURREHMAN	ABIDA
ABDULHAMEED	ABDUS	ABIDAH
ABDULHAMID	ABDUS-SAMAD	ABIDEEN
ABDULILAH	ABDUS-SAMI	ABIDEMI
ABDULJABBAR	ABDUSALAM	ABIDUL
ABDULKADER	ABDUSSALAM	ABIDUR
ABDULKADIR	ABDUSSAMAD	ABIE
ABDULKAREEM	ABE	ABIEL
ABDULKARIM	ABED	ABIEYUWA
ABDULKHALIQ	ABEDA	ABIGAEL
ABDULLA	ABEED	ABIGAIL
ABDULLAAH	ABEEDA	ABIGAIL-LOUISE
ABDULLAAHI	ABEEDAH	ABIGAIL-ROSE
ABDULLAH	ABEEHA	ABIGAILE
ABDULLAHI	ABEEL	ABIGALE
ABDULLATEEF	ABEER	ABIGAYLE
ABDULLATIF	ABEERA	ABIGEL
ABDULLOH	ABEERAH	ABIHA
ABDULMAJEED	ABEL	ABIJAH
ABDULMAJID	ABELA	ABIJOT
ABDULMALEK	ABELLA	ABILASH
ABDULMALIK	ABEN	ABILENE
ABDULMUIZZ	ABENA	ABIMBOLA
ABDULQADIR	ABENEZER	ABINA
ABDULRAHEEM	ABENI	ABINAASH
ABDULRAHIM	ABHAY	ABINASH
ABDULRAHMAN	ABHI	ABINAYA
ABDULREHMAN	ABHIA	ABINAYAN
ABDULRHMAN	ABHIJAY	ABINESH
ABDULSALAM	ABHIJEET	ABIODUN
ABDULSAMAD	ABHIJIT	ABIOLA
ABDULWAHAB	ABHIJITH	ABIONA
ABDULWAHHAB	ABHIJOT	ABIR
ABDULWAHID	ABHIMANYU	ABIRA

ABIRAJ
ABIRAMI
ABIRAMY
ABISAN
ABISHA
ABISHAI
ABISHAKE
ABISHAN
ABISHANTH
ABISHEK
ABISOLA
ABISOYE
ABITHA
ABITHAN
ABIYA
ABIZER
ABLA
ABNER
ABOU
ABOUBACAR
ABOUBAKAR
ABRA
ABRAAR
ABRAHAM
ABRAHIM
ABRAM
ABRAR
ABRIANNA
ABRIEL
ABRIELLA
ABRIELLE
ABRIL
ABRISH
ABSAR
ABSHIR
ABU
ABU-BAKAR
ABU-BAKR
ABU-HURAIRA
ABU-SUFYAN
ABUBACARR
ABUBAKAR
ABUBAKARR
ABUBAKER
ABUBAKKAR
ABUBAKR
ABUHURAIRAH
ABUKAR
ABUL
ABUZAR
ABY
ABYAAN
ABYAD
ABYAN
ABYGAIL
ABYGAYLE
ACACIA
ACE
ACELYA
ACER
ACEY
ACHILLE
ACHILLEAS
ACHILLES
ACHINTYA
ACHRAF
ACHSA
ACHSAH
ACKEEM
ADA
ADA-GRACE
ADA-MAY
ADA-ROSE
ADAAM
ADABELLE
ADAEZE
ADAH
ADAIR
ADAL
ADALIA
ADALIE
ADALIND
ADALINE
ADALYN
ADALYNN
ADAM
ADAM-JAMES
ADAM-JUNIOR
ADAMA
ADAMAS
ADAMO
ADAMS
ADAN
ADANA
ADANNA
ADAOBI
ADAORA
ADAR
ADARA
ADARSH
ADAS
ADAUGO
ADAYA
ADDAI
ADDALYN
ADDAM
ADDIE
ADDIEN
ADDIENA
ADDILYN
ADDIS
ADDISON
ADDISYN
ADDYSON
ADE
ADEA
ADEANA
ADEBAYO
ADEBISI
ADEBOLA
ADEBOWALE
ADEBOYE
ADEDAMOLA
ADEDAPO
ADEDAYO
ADEDEJI
ADEDOLAPO
ADEDOTUN
ADEDOYIN
ADEE
ADEEB
ADEEBA
ADEEBAH
ADEEL
ADEELA
ADEEM
ADEEN
ADEENA
ADEESA
ADEEVA
ADEKEMI
ADEKUNLE
ADEL
ADELA

ADELAIDE	ADHAM	ADNAAN
ADELE	ADHAVAN	ADNAN
ADELEKE	ADHEEM	ADOM
ADELIA	ADHEEN	ADOMAS
ADELIE	ADHIRA	ADON
ADELIN	ADHIRAJ	ADONA
ADELINA	ADHNAN	ADONAI
ADELINE	ADHRIT	ADONAY
ADELL	ADHVAITH	ADONIA
ADELLA	ADHVIK	ADONIJAH
ADELLE	ADHYA	ADONIS
ADELYN	ADI	ADORA
ADELYNN	ADIA	ADREES
ADEM	ADIAN	ADRIA
ADEMAYOWA	ADIB	ADRIAAN
ADEMIDE	ADIBA	ADRIAN
ADEMOLA	ADIBAH	ADRIANA
ADEN	ADIE	ADRIANAS
ADENA	ADIEL	ADRIANE
ADENIKE	ADIFAAH	ADRIANNA
ADENIYI	ADIL	ADRIANNE
ADEOLA	ADILA	ADRIANO
ADEOLU	ADILAH	ADRIANS
ADEOLUWA	ADILSON	ADRIATIK
ADEPEJU	ADIN	ADRIEL
ADEREMI	ADINA	ADRIELLE
ADERINOLA	ADIRA	ADRIEN
ADERINSOLA	ADISA	ADRIENNE
ADERONKE	ADISON	ADRIJA
ADERYN	ADIT	ADRIJANA
ADESEWA	ADITH	ADRIJUS
ADESH	ADITHI	ADRIKA
ADESIRE	ADITHYA	ADRIN
ADESOLA	ADITI	ADRINA
ADESUWA	ADITRI	ADRIS
ADETAYO	ADITYA	ADRITA
ADETOKUNBO	ADIVA	ADSHAYAN
ADETOLA	ADIY	ADUNOLA
ADETOMIWA	ADIYA	ADVAIT
ADETOUN	ADIYAAN	ADVAITA
ADETUNJI	ADIYAN	ADVAITH
ADETUTU	ADJA	ADVAY
ADEWALE	ADJOA	ADVIK
ADEWONUOLA	ADLANE	ADVIKA
ADEWUMI	ADLER	ADVIT
ADEWUNMI	ADLEY	ADVITA
ADEYEMI	ADN	ADVITH
ADEYINKA	ADNA	ADWIN

ADWOA
ADY
ADYA
ADYAAN
ADYAN
AEDAN
AEDDAN
AEDEN
AEESHA
AEISHA
AELA
AELFRED
AELLA
AEMAN
AEMELIA
AEMILIA
AENEAS
AENGUS
AEON
AERIN
AERIS
AERITH
AERON
AERONA
AERYN
AESHA
AESON
AEVA
AEVAH
AEYSHA
AFAAF
AFAAN
AFAF
AFAN
AFAQ
AFEEF
AFEEFA
AFEEFAH
AFET
AFFAAN
AFFAF
AFFAN
AFFIA
AFIA
AFIFA
AFIFAH
AFIQ
AFIRA
AFIYA
AFIYAH
AFIZAH
AFJOL
AFNAAN
AFNAN
AFOLABI
AFOLARIN
AFON
AFONSO
AFRA
AFRAA
AFRAH
AFRAZ
AFREEN
AFRICA
AFRIDA
AFRIKA
AFRIN
AFRINA
AFRUZA
AFSA
AFSAH
AFSANA
AFSAR
AFSARA
AFSEEN
AFSHA
AFSHAH
AFSHAN
AFSHANA
AFSHEEN
AFTAB
AFTON
AFUA
AFZA
AFZAAL
AFZAL
AGAM
AGAMBIR
AGAMDEEP
AGAMJOT
AGAMPREET
AGAMVEER
AGAPE
AGASTHYA
AGASTYA
AGATA
AGATHA
AGATHE
AGGELIKI
AGGIE
AGHA
AGIM
AGIT
AGNE
AGNES
AGNESA
AGNESE
AGNIESZKA
AGNIUS
AGON
AGOTA
AGRIM
AGRON
AGUSTIN
AHAAN
AHAANA
AHAB
AHAD
AHAMED
AHAN
AHANA
AHARAN
AHARON
AHCENE
AHDIA
AHEED
AHIL
AHLAAM
AHLAAN
AHLAM
AHLAN
AHMAD
AHMAD-RAZA
AHMADOU
AHMAR
AHMED
AHMED-RAZA
AHMER
AHMET
AHNAF
AHREN
AHRON
AHSAAN
AHSAN

AHSANUL	AILIS	AISA
AHSEN	AILISE	AISEA
AHTISHAM	AILISH	AISHA
AHTSHAM	AILISHA	AISHAH
AHUVA	AILLA	AISHANI
AHYAAN	AILSA	AISHAT
AHYAN	AIMA	AISHATU
AI	AIMAH	AISHI
AIA	AIMAL	AISHIA
AIAN	AIMAN	AISHLEEN
AIBHLIN	AIMAR	AISHLING
AIBHLINN	AIME	AISHPREET
AICHA	AIMEE	AISHWARYA
AIDA	AIMEE-	AISLA
AIDAAN	AIMEE-GRACE	AISLEYNE
AIDAH	AIMEE-JANE	AISLIN
AIDAN	AIMEE-JAYNE	AISLING
AIDAN-JAMES	AIMEE-JO	AISLINN
AIDAS	AIMEE-LEA	AISOSA
AIDEEN	AIMEE-LEE	AISSA
AIDEL	AIMEE-LEIGH	AISSATA
AIDEN	AIMEE-LOUISE	AISSATOU
AIDEN-JAMES	AIMEE-MAE	AISTE
AIDEN-JAY	AIMEE-MAY	AISTIS
AIDEN-LEE	AIMEE-ROSE	AISWARYA
AIDON	AIMEN	AISYA
AIDY	AIMI	AISYAH
AIDYN	AIMIE	AITANA
AIELA	AIMIEE	AITOR
AIESHA	AIMUN	AIVA
AIFE	AIMY	AIVA-ROSE
AIHAM	AIN	AIVAH
AIJAZ	AINA	AIVARAS
AIKA	AINARA	AIYA
AIKAM	AINE	AIYAAN
AIKATERINI	AINHOA	AIYAH
AIKEN	AINI	AIYAN
AIKO	AINSLEIGH	AIYANA
AILA	AINSLEY	AIYANAH
AILAH	AINSLIE	AIYANNA
AILAN	AIRA	AIYAT
AILANI	AIRAH	AIYAZ
AILBE	AIREN	AIYESHA
AILBHE	AIRI	AIYLA
AILEEN	AIRIDAS	AIYLAH
AILIDH	AIRLIE	AIYSHA
AILIE	AIRON	AIYUSH
AILIN	AIRONAS	AIYZA

AIYZAH
AIZA
AIZAH
AIZAH-NOOR
AIZEN
AIZZA
AIZZAH
AJ
AJA
AJAI
AJAIB
AJAN
AJANA
AJANI
AJANTHAN
AJAX
AJAY
AJAZ
AJEET
AJESH
AJHAR
AJI
AJIBOLA
AJIT
AJLA
AJMAL
AJOONI
AJUNI
AJUS
AJWA
AJWAD
AJWAH
AKAAL
AKAALDEEP
AKAASH
AKACHUKWU
AKAI
AKAIN
AKAL
AKAM
AKAN
AKANE
AKANKSHA
AKAR
AKARAN
AKARI
AKARSH
AKASH

AKASHA
AKASHDEEP
AKASYA
AKAY
AKAYLA
AKAYSHA
AKBAR
AKBER
AKEAL
AKEEB
AKEEL
AKEELA
AKEELAH
AKEEM
AKEIN
AKEIRA
AKEISHA
AKEMI
AKHEEL
AKHIL
AKHIRA
AKHLAQ
AKHSA
AKHTAR
AKI
AKIA
AKIB
AKIDA
AKIEL
AKIERA
AKIESHA
AKIF
AKIFA
AKIFAH
AKIKUR
AKIL
AKILA
AKILAH
AKIM
AKIN
AKINA
AKINLOLU
AKINOLA
AKINTAYO
AKINTOMIWA
AKINTUNDE
AKINYEMI
AKIO

AKIRA
AKIRAH
AKISHA
AKITO
AKIVA
AKLIMA
AKMAL
AKOREDE
AKOS
AKOSUA
AKRAM
AKRITI
AKSA
AKSAA
AKSAH
AKSARA
AKSAYAN
AKSEL
AKSH
AKSHA
AKSHAJ
AKSHAN
AKSHANA
AKSHAR
AKSHARA
AKSHARAA
AKSHARAN
AKSHAT
AKSHATA
AKSHATH
AKSHAY
AKSHAYA
AKSHAYAA
AKSHAYAH
AKSHAYAN
AKSHAYE
AKSHAYEN
AKSHIT
AKSHITA
AKSHITH
AKUA
AKVILE
AKWASI
AL
AL-AMEEN
AL-AMIN
AL-YASA
ALA

ALA'A
ALAA
ALAANA
ALABAMA
ALAE
ALAGIE
ALAHNA
ALAIA
ALAIA-MAI
ALAIBA
ALAIKA
ALAIN
ALAINA
ALAINE
ALAIYA
ALAIYAH
ALAIYNA
ALAIZA
ALAM
ALAMEEN
ALAMIN
ALAN
ALANA
ALANA-MAE
ALANA-RAE
ALANA-ROSE
ALANAH
ALANAS
ALAND
ALANI
ALANIA
ALANIS
ALANNA
ALANNAH
ALANNAH-MAE
ALANNAH-ROSE
ALANNIS
ALANOOD
ALANOUD
ALANS
ALANTA
ALANTIS
ALANYA
ALANYAH
ALARA
ALARAH
ALARIA
ALARIC

ALARIK
ALARNA
ALARNAH
ALARNI
ALARNIE
ALASDAIR
ALASIA
ALASKA
ALASTAIR
ALATHEA
ALAURA
ALAW
ALAYA
ALAYAH
ALAYAH-MAE
ALAYAH-ROSE
ALAYHA
ALAYLA
ALAYNA
ALAYNAH
ALAYSIA
ALAZAR
ALBA
ALBA-ROSE
ALBAN
ALBANE
ALBANO
ALBANY
ALBARA
ALBARAA
ALBATOOL
ALBE
ALBEE
ALBERT
ALBERT-JOE
ALBERTA
ALBERTINE
ALBERTO
ALBEY
ALBI
ALBIE
ALBIE-GEORGE
ALBIE-JAMES
ALBIE-JAY
ALBIE-JOE
ALBIE-LEE
ALBIN
ALBINA

ALBION
ALBIONA
ALBORZ
ALBUS
ALBY
ALDEN
ALDIN
ALDION
ALDO
ALDOUS
ALDRICH
ALDRIN
ALDWIN
ALEA
ALEACIA
ALEAH
ALEAHA
ALEANA
ALEASHA
ALEC
ALECHANDRO
ALECIA
ALECK
ALECSANDER
ALED
ALEEA
ALEEAH
ALEECE
ALEECIA
ALEEHA
ALEEM
ALEEMA
ALEEMAH
ALEEN
ALEENA
ALEENAH
ALEESA
ALEESHA
ALEESHBA
ALEEYA
ALEEYAH
ALEEZA
ALEEZAH
ALEEZAY
ALEGRA
ALEGRIA
ALEHA
ALEHANDRO

ALEIA
ALEIAH
ALEIGHA
ALEIGHA-MAE
ALEIGHSHA
ALEINA
ALEISHA
ALEIYA
ALEJANDRA
ALEJANDRO
ALEK
ALEKH
ALEKS
ALEKSA
ALEKSANDAR
ALEKSANDER
ALEKSANDR
ALEKSANDRA
ALEKSANDRAS
ALEKSANDRS
ALEKSAS
ALEKSEI
ALEKSEJ
ALEKSEJS
ALEKSEY
ALEKSI
ALEKSIA
ALEKSIS
ALEKSS
ALEKSY
ALEM
ALEMA
ALEN
ALENA
ALEND
ALENNA
ALENS
ALERO
ALES
ALESANDRO
ALESHA
ALESHA-MAE
ALESHA-MARIE
ALESHA-ROSE
ALESHIA
ALESI
ALESIA
ALESIO
ALESKA
ALESSA
ALESSANDRA
ALESSANDRO
ALESSI
ALESSIA
ALESSIA-MARIA
ALESSIO
ALESSYA
ALETA
ALETHEA
ALETHEIA
ALETHIA
ALETIA
ALETTA
ALEV
ALEX
ALEX-JAMES
ALEX-JAY
ALEX-JUNIOR
ALEXA
ALEXA-LEIGH
ALEXA-MAE
ALEXA-MAY
ALEXA-ROSE
ALEXAH
ALEXANDA
ALEXANDAR
ALEXANDER
ALEXANDER-JAMES
ALEXANDR
ALEXANDRA
ALEXANDRE
ALEXANDREA
ALEXANDRIA
ALEXANDRINA
ALEXANDRO
ALEXANDROS
ALEXANDRU
ALEXAS
ALEXAVIER
ALEXCIA
ALEXEI
ALEXEY
ALEXI
ALEXIA
ALEXIA-LEIGH
ALEXIA-MAE
ALEXIA-MAY
ALEXIA-ROSE
ALEXIAH
ALEXIE
ALEXINA
ALEXINE
ALEXIOS
ALEXIS
ALEXIS-JADE
ALEXIS-LEIGH
ALEXIS-LOUISE
ALEXIS-MAE
ALEXIS-MARIE
ALEXIS-MAY
ALEXIS-ROSE
ALEXIYA
ALEXSANDER
ALEXSANDRA
ALEXSI
ALEXSIS
ALEXUS
ALEXXA
ALEXY
ALEXYS
ALEXZANDER
ALEXZANDRA
ALEYA
ALEYAH
ALEYNA
ALEYSHA
ALF
ALFEE
ALFEY
ALFFI
ALFFIE
ALFI
ALFIE
ALFIE-
ALFIE-DEAN
ALFIE-GEORGE
ALFIE-J
ALFIE-JACK
ALFIE-JAI
ALFIE-JAMES
ALFIE-JAY
ALFIE-JOE
ALFIE-JOHN
ALFIE-JOSEPH

ALFIE-JUNIOR	ALICIA-MAE	ALISHA-MAI
ALFIE-LEE	ALICIA-MARIE	ALISHA-MARIE
ALFIE-PAUL	ALICIA-MAY	ALISHA-MAY
ALFIE-RAY	ALICIA-ROSE	ALISHA-ROSE
ALFIE-RYAN	ALICJA	ALISHAA
ALFIE-THOMAS	ALICK	ALISHABA
ALFIE-WILLIAM	ALIDA	ALISHAH
ALFIEE	ALIDIA	ALISHAN
ALFIN	ALIE	ALISHBA
ALFIO	ALIEA	ALISHBAH
ALFIYA	ALIENA	ALISHEA
ALFONSO	ALIENOR	ALISHER
ALFRED	ALIESHA	ALISHIA
ALFREDO	ALIEU	ALISHMA
ALFY	ALIF	ALISHYA
ALGERNON	ALIFA	ALISIA
ALHAGIE	ALIFIYA	ALISIJA
ALHAJI	ALIHA	ALISINA
ALHASAN	ALIHAN	ALISIYA
ALHASSAN	ALIJAH	ALISON
ALHENA	ALIKA	ALISSA
ALI	ALIKI	ALISSA-MAE
ALI-ABBAS	ALILA	ALISSE
ALI-AKBAR	ALILAH	ALISSIA
ALI-HASSAN	ALILIA	ALISSIYA
ALI-RAZA	ALIM	ALISSON
ALIA	ALIMA	ALISSYA
ALIAA	ALIMAH	ALISTAIR
ALIABBAS	ALIMAT	ALISTAR
ALIAH	ALIN	ALISTER
ALIAKBAR	ALINA	ALISYA
ALIANA	ALINAH	ALITA
ALIANNA	ALINE	ALIVIA
ALIANNAH	ALINNA	ALIVIA-LEIGH
ALIAS	ALIONA	ALIVIA-ROSE
ALICA	ALIOU	ALIVIAH
ALICAN	ALIOUNE	ALIX
ALICE	ALIREZA	ALIXANDER
ALICE-ANN	ALIS	ALIXANDRA
ALICE-JANE	ALISA	ALIYA
ALICE-LOUISE	ALISAH	ALIYAAN
ALICE-MAE	ALISAN	ALIYAH
ALICE-MARIE	ALISCIA	ALIYAH-GRACE
ALICE-MAY	ALISDAIR	ALIYAH-MAE
ALICE-ROSE	ALISE	ALIYAH-ROSE
ALICEA	ALISHA	ALIYAN
ALICIA	ALISHA-LEIGH	ALIYANA
ALICIA-GRACE	ALISHA-MAE	ALIYAT

ALIYE	ALLISHA	ALPHONSA
ALIYHA	ALLISIA	ALPHONSE
ALIYSHA	ALLISON	ALPHONSO
ALIYU	ALLISSA	ALPHONSUS
ALIYYA	ALLISSIA	ALPHY
ALIYYAH	ALLISTAIR	ALREEM
ALIYZA	ALLISTER	ALROY
ALIZ	ALLIYA	ALSTON
ALIZA	ALLIYAH	ALTAF
ALIZA-MAE	ALLORA	ALTAIR
ALIZA-RAE	ALLY	ALTAN
ALIZAH	ALLYA	ALTAY
ALIZAY	ALLYSA	ALTEO
ALIZE	ALLYSHA	ALTHEA
ALIZEE	ALLYSIA	ALTIN
ALIZEH	ALLYSON	ALTINA
ALIZEY	ALLYSSA	ALTON
ALJAWHARA	ALLYSSIA	ALUN
ALJAWHARAH	ALMA	ALUNA
ALKA	ALMAAN	ALURA
ALKETA	ALMAAS	ALUSINE
ALLA	ALMAMY	ALVA
ALLAM	ALMAN	ALVAN
ALLAN	ALMAS	ALVAR
ALLANA	ALMAZ	ALVARO
ALLANAH	ALMEER	ALVEENA
ALLANAH-ROSE	ALMEERA	ALVEERA
ALLANNA	ALMINA	ALVEY
ALLANNAH	ALMIR	ALVI
ALLANYA	ALMIRA	ALVIA
ALLARNA	ALOK	ALVIE
ALLAYA	ALOKA	ALVIN
ALLAYAH	ALOM	ALVINA
ALLE	ALOMA	ALVIRA
ALLEAH	ALON	ALVIS
ALLEGRA	ALONA	ALVY
ALLEN	ALONDRA	ALVYN
ALLENA	ALONIAB	ALWALEED
ALLESSE	ALONSO	ALWIN
ALLEX	ALONZO	ALWYN
ALLEXIS	ALORA	ALY
ALLEYAH	ALOYSIUS	ALYA
ALLI	ALP	ALYAAN
ALLIA	ALPER	ALYAANAH
ALLIAH	ALPEREN	ALYAH
ALLIANA	ALPHA	ALYAN
ALLICIA	ALPHIE	ALYANA
ALLIE	ALPHONS	ALYANNA

ALYAS
ALYCE
ALYCEE
ALYCIA
ALYDIA
ALYESHA
ALYIA
ALYIAH
ALYISHA
ALYISSIA
ALYLAH
ALYN
ALYNA
ALYONA
ALYRA
ALYS
ALYSA
ALYSCIA
ALYSE
ALYSHA
ALYSHEA
ALYSHIA
ALYSIA
ALYSON
ALYSS
ALYSSA
ALYSSA-JADE
ALYSSA-MAE
ALYSSA-MAY
ALYSSA-ROSE
ALYSSE
ALYSSIA
ALYSSIA-MAE
ALYSSIA-ROSE
ALYSSYA
ALYVIA
ALYX
ALYXANDRA
ALYZA
ALYZAH
ALYZZA
ALZAHRA
ALZBETA
AMA
AMAAD
AMAAIMA
AMAAL
AMAAN
AMAANA
AMAANAH
AMAANI
AMAAR
AMAARA
AMAARAH
AMAAYA
AMAAZ
AMABEL
AMABELLE
AMAD
AMADEO
AMADEUS
AMADEUSZ
AMADOU
AMADU
AMAIA
AMAIAH
AMAIMA
AMAIRA
AMAIRAH
AMAIYA
AMAIYAH
AMAKA
AMAL
AMALA
AMALEA
AMALEE
AMALEIGH
AMALI
AMALIA
AMALIAH
AMALIE
AMALIE-ROSE
AMALYA
AMAMA
AMAN
AMANA
AMANAH
AMANAT
AMANDA
AMANDEEP
AMANDINE
AMANDIP
AMANI
AMANIE
AMANITA
AMANIYA
AMANJEET
AMANJIT
AMANJOT
AMANN
AMANPREET
AMANRAJ
AMANUEL
AMANULLAH
AMANVEER
AMANVIR
AMANY
AMAR
AMARA
AMARA-ROSE
AMARACHI
AMARACHUKWU
AMARAH
AMARDEEP
AMARE
AMAREE
AMARI
AMARIA
AMARIAH
AMARIE
AMARII
AMARIO
AMARION
AMARIS
AMARISA
AMARISE
AMARISSA
AMARIYAH
AMARJEET
AMARJIT
AMARJOT
AMARLEEN
AMARLIA
AMARN
AMARNI
AMARNIE
AMARO
AMARPAL
AMARPREET
AMARRI
AMARU
AMARVEER
AMARVIR
AMARYLLIS

AMATUL
AMATULLAH
AMAURI
AMAURY
AMAY
AMAYA
AMAYA-RAE
AMAYA-ROSE
AMAYAH
AMAYRA
AMAYRAH
AMAZIAH
AMAZON
AMBA
AMBAH
AMBAR
AMBER
AMBER-
AMBER-GRACE
AMBER-JADE
AMBER-JANE
AMBER-JAYNE
AMBER-JO
AMBER-LEA
AMBER-LEE
AMBER-LEIGH
AMBER-LILLY
AMBER-LILY
AMBER-LOUISE
AMBER-MAE
AMBER-MARIE
AMBER-MAY
AMBER-RAE
AMBER-ROSE
AMBEREEN
AMBERLEA
AMBERLEIGH
AMBERLEY
AMBERLIE
AMBERLY
AMBIA
AMBIKA
AMBIYA
AMBRA
AMBRE
AMBREEN
AMBRIN
AMBROSE

AMBROSIA
AMBUR
AME
AMEA
AMEALIA
AMED
AMEDEEA
AMEDEO
AMEE
AMEELA
AMEELAH
AMEELIA
AMEEMA
AMEEN
AMEENA
AMEENAH
AMEER
AMEERA
AMEERAH
AMEERAT
AMEESHA
AMEILA
AMEILIA
AMEIRA
AMEL
AMELA
AMELEA
AMELEAH
AMELI
AMELIA
AMELIA-
AMELIA-ALICE
AMELIA-ANN
AMELIA-ANNE
AMELIA-BROOKE
AMELIA-ELIZABETH
AMELIA-FAITH
AMELIA-FAYE
AMELIA-GRACE
AMELIA-HOPE
AMELIA-JADE
AMELIA-JANE
AMELIA-JAYDE
AMELIA-JAYNE
AMELIA-JEAN
AMELIA-JO
AMELIA-LEE
AMELIA-LEIGH

AMELIA-LILLIE
AMELIA-LILLY
AMELIA-LILY
AMELIA-LOUISE
AMELIA-MAE
AMELIA-MAI
AMELIA-MARIE
AMELIA-MAY
AMELIA-PAIGE
AMELIA-RAE
AMELIA-ROSE
AMELIA-SKYE
AMELIAH
AMELIAH-ROSE
AMELIE
AMELIE-GRACE
AMELIE-MAE
AMELIE-MAI
AMELIE-ROSE
AMELIJA
AMELINA
AMELINE
AMELIO
AMELIYA
AMELIYAH
AMELJA
AMELLE
AMELLIA
AMELLIE
AMELY
AMELYA
AMEN
AMENA
AMENAH
AMENZE
AMER
AMERA
AMERAH
AMERIA
AMERIE
AMETHYST
AMEY
AMEYA
AMEZ
AMI
AMI-LEIGH
AMI-LOUISE
AMIA

AMIAH	AMINUR	AMOUR
AMIAS	AMIR	AMOY
AMICA	AMIRA	AMOYA
AMICIA	AMIRA-ROSE	AMR
AMICIE	AMIRAH	AMRA
AMID	AMIRALI	AMRAH
AMIDAT	AMIRAT	AMRAIZ
AMIE	AMIRUL	AMRAJ
AMIE-LEE	AMISA	AMRAN
AMIE-LEIGH	AMISH	AMREECE
AMIE-LOUISE	AMISHA	AMREEN
AMIEE	AMISHI	AMREENA
AMIEE-LEIGH	AMIT	AMREET
AMIEE-LOUISE	AMITA	AMREETA
AMIEL	AMITAI	AMRIA
AMIELEIGH	AMITIS	AMRIK
AMIELIA	AMITOJ	AMRIN
AMIERA	AMITY	AMRINA
AMII	AMIYA	AMRINDER
AMIIN	AMIYAH	AMRIT
AMIINA	AMIYAH-ROSE	AMRITA
AMIIR	AMJAD	AMRITHA
AMIIRA	AMJED	AMRITPAL
AMIKA	AMJID	AMRITPREET
AMIL	AMMA	AMRO
AMILA	AMMAAR	AMROM
AMILAH	AMMAARA	AMRUTHA
AMILEA	AMMAARAH	AMRY
AMILEAH	AMMAD	AMTUL
AMILEE	AMMAL	AMULYA
AMILEIGH	AMMAN	AMUN
AMILIA	AMMAR	AMY
AMILIE	AMMARA	AMY-
AMILLIA	AMMARAH	AMY-ANN
AMILLIE	AMMIE	AMY-BETH
AMILY	AMNA	AMY-GRACE
AMILYA	AMNAH	AMY-JADE
AMIMA	AMNEEK	AMY-JANE
AMIN	AMNEET	AMY-JAYNE
AMINA	AMOGH	AMY-JO
AMINAH	AMOL	AMY-LEA
AMINAH-NOOR	AMON	AMY-LEE
AMINAT	AMOR	AMY-LEIGH
AMINATA	AMORA	AMY-LOU
AMINE	AMORAE	AMY-LOUISE
AMINOOR	AMORE	AMY-MAE
AMINTA	AMORY	AMY-MARIE
AMINUL	AMOS	AMY-MAY

AMY-RAE	ANAISS	ANDALEEB
AMY-ROSE	ANAIYA	ANDER
AMYA	ANAIYAH	ANDERS
AMYAH	ANAKIN	ANDERSON
AMYE	ANALEIGH	ANDI
AMYLEA	ANALEISE	ANDIA
AMYLEE	ANALIESE	ANDIE
AMYLEIGH	ANALISA	ANDILE
AMYLIA	ANALISE	ANDOR
AMYLOUISE	ANALUCIA	ANDRA
AMYMA	ANAM	ANDRADA
AMYRA	ANAMARIA	ANDRAE
AMYRAH	ANAMIKA	ANDRAS
AMZA	ANAMTA	ANDRE
AN	ANAN	ANDRE-JUNIOR
ANA	ANAND	ANDREA
ANA-LUCIA	ANANDA	ANDREANA
ANA-MARIA	ANANDI	ANDREANNA
ANA-SOFIA	ANANNYA	ANDREAS
ANAAYA	ANANT	ANDREEA
ANAAYAH	ANANTH	ANDREI
ANAB	ANANYA	ANDREIA
ANABEL	ANANYAA	ANDREJ
ANABELA	ANARA	ANDREJA
ANABELL	ANARITA	ANDREJS
ANABELLA	ANAS	ANDRES
ANABELLE	ANASHE	ANDREW
ANABETH	ANASS	ANDREW-JAMES
ANABIA	ANASTACIA	ANDREW-JOHN
ANABIAH	ANASTASIA	ANDREW-JUNIOR
ANABIYA	ANASTASIJA	ANDREY
ANABIYAH	ANASTASIOS	ANDREYA
ANAE	ANASTASIYA	ANDRI
ANAELLE	ANASTAZIA	ANDRIA
ANAGHA	ANASTAZJA	ANDRIANA
ANAH	ANATOLE	ANDRIANNA
ANAHI	ANAUM	ANDRIES
ANAHID	ANAY	ANDRINA
ANAHITA	ANAYA	ANDRIUS
ANAI	ANAYAA	ANDRIY
ANAIA	ANAYAH	ANDROMEDA
ANAIAH	ANAYAH-ROSE	ANDROULLA
ANAIKA	ANAYS	ANDRZEJ
ANAIS	ANAYSS	ANDUENA
ANAIS-ROSE	ANBAR	ANDY
ANAISA	ANCA	ANDZELIKA
ANAISE	ANCHAL	ANE
ANAISHA	ANDA	ANEA

ANEEK	ANGE	ANICA
ANEEKA	ANGEL	ANIELA
ANEEKAH	ANGEL-GRACE	ANIELLA
ANEEKHA	ANGEL-HOPE	ANIESHA
ANEEL	ANGEL-LEIGH	ANIK
ANEELA	ANGEL-LOUISE	ANIKA
ANEEQ	ANGEL-MAE	ANIKAH
ANEEQA	ANGEL-MAI	ANIKE
ANEEQAH	ANGEL-MARIE	ANIKET
ANEES	ANGEL-MAY	ANIL
ANEESA	ANGEL-ROSE	ANILA
ANEESAH	ANGELA	ANILAH
ANEESH	ANGELE	ANINA
ANEESHA	ANGELEE	ANIQ
ANEET	ANGELEEN	ANIQA
ANEEYA	ANGELENA	ANIQAH
ANEEZA	ANGELENE	ANIQUE
ANEIL	ANGELI	ANIR
ANEIRA	ANGELIA	ANIRUDDHA
ANEIRIN	ANGELIC	ANIRUDH
ANEISHA	ANGELICA	ANIS
ANEKA	ANGELICA-ROSE	ANISA
ANEL	ANGELIE	ANISAH
ANELA	ANGELIKA	ANISE
ANELIA	ANGELIKI	ANISH
ANELISE	ANGELIN	ANISHA
ANELKA	ANGELINA	ANISHAH
ANES	ANGELINE	ANISHKA
ANESA	ANGELIQUE	ANISIA
ANESH	ANGELISE	ANISS
ANESHA	ANGELL	ANISSA
ANESHKA	ANGELLE	ANISUL
ANESS	ANGELO	ANISUR
ANESSA	ANGELOS	ANITA
ANEST	ANGELPREET	ANITHA
ANESU	ANGELUS	ANITRA
ANETA	ANGELYN	ANIV
ANETTA	ANGHARAD	ANIYA
ANETTE	ANGIE	ANIYAH
ANEURIN	ANGLIA	ANIYAH-RAE
ANEYA	ANGUS	ANIYAH-ROSE
ANEZKA	ANH	ANIZA
ANFA	ANHA	ANJA
ANFAAL	ANHAD	ANJALEE
ANFAL	ANHAR	ANJALI
ANFISA	ANI	ANJANA
ANGAD	ANIA	ANJANI
ANGADVEER	ANIAH	ANJAY

ANJE	ANNAH	ANNETTA
ANJELI	ANNAIS	ANNETTE
ANJELICA	ANNAIYA	ANNI
ANJELINA	ANNAIYAH	ANNIA
ANJESA	ANNAKAY	ANNIAH
ANJIKA	ANNALEA	ANNICA
ANJLEE	ANNALEASE	ANNICE
ANJLI	ANNALEE	ANNIE
ANJOLA	ANNALEECE	ANNIE-GRACE
ANJOLAOLUWA	ANNALEESE	ANNIE-LOU
ANJU	ANNALEIGH	ANNIE-LOUISE
ANJULI	ANNALEISE	ANNIE-MAE
ANJUM	ANNALENA	ANNIE-MAI
ANJUMA	ANNALESE	ANNIE-MARIE
ANJUMAN	ANNALIA	ANNIE-MAY
ANKE	ANNALIE	ANNIE-RAE
ANKIT	ANNALIESE	ANNIE-ROSE
ANKITA	ANNALISA	ANNIJA
ANKUR	ANNALISE	ANNIKA
ANKUSH	ANNALISSE	ANNIS
ANMOL	ANNALIZE	ANNISA
ANN	ANNALYSE	ANNISE
ANN-MARIE	ANNAM	ANNISHA
ANNA	ANNAMAE	ANNISSA
ANNA-	ANNAMARIA	ANNIYA
ANNA-BELLA	ANNAMARIE	ANNIYAH
ANNA-LEE	ANNAMAY	ANNMARIA
ANNA-LEIGH	ANNAN	ANNMARIE
ANNA-LENA	ANNANYA	ANNMARY
ANNA-LISA	ANNAROSE	ANNORA
ANNA-LISE	ANNAS	ANNUM
ANNA-LOUISE	ANNASTASIA	ANNY
ANNA-LUCIA	ANNAYA	ANNYA
ANNA-MAE	ANNAYAH	ANNYS
ANNA-MAI	ANNE	ANOJAN
ANNA-MARIA	ANNE-MARIE	ANOKH
ANNA-MARIE	ANNEKA	ANOKHI
ANNA-MAY	ANNEKE	ANOLA
ANNA-ROSE	ANNELI	ANONA
ANNA-SOPHIA	ANNELIE	ANOOP
ANNABEL	ANNELIES	ANOOSH
ANNABEL-ROSE	ANNELIESE	ANOOSHA
ANNABELL	ANNELISE	ANORA
ANNABELLA	ANNELLE	ANOSH
ANNABELLA-ROSE	ANNEMARIE	ANOSHA
ANNABELLE	ANNES	ANOTIDA
ANNABELLE-ROSE	ANNESHA	ANOTIDAISHE
ANNABETH	ANNEST	ANOTIDASHE

ANOUAR
ANOUK
ANOUSCHKA
ANOUSH
ANOUSHA
ANOUSHEH
ANOUSHKA
ANOUSKA
ANQI
ANRAJ
ANS
ANSA
ANSAAR
ANSAH
ANSAM
ANSAR
ANSEL
ANSELM
ANSH
ANSHA
ANSHARAH
ANSHDEEP
ANSHI
ANSHIKA
ANSHITA
ANSHPREET
ANSHU
ANSHUL
ANSHVEER
ANSON
ANTANAS
ANTARA
ANTEK
ANTHEA
ANTHI
ANTHONIA
ANTHONIE
ANTHONY
ANTHONY-JAMES
ANTHONY-JOHN
ANTHONY-JUNIOR
ANTIGONE
ANTIGONI
ANTOINE
ANTOINETTE
ANTON
ANTONELLA
ANTONETTE

ANTONI
ANTONIA
ANTONIA-MARIA
ANTONIE
ANTONIETTA
ANTONIN
ANTONINA
ANTONINO
ANTONIO
ANTONIOS
ANTONIS
ANTONY
ANTOSIA
ANTWAN
ANTWON
ANTWONE
ANU
ANUAR
ANUJ
ANUJA
ANUJAN
ANUJIN
ANUKSHA
ANUM
ANUOLUWA
ANUOLUWAPO
ANURAG
ANUREET
ANUSAN
ANUSH
ANUSHA
ANUSHAN
ANUSHKA
ANUSHREE
ANUSHRI
ANVAY
ANVI
ANVIKA
ANVITA
ANVITHA
ANWAAR
ANWAR
ANWEN
ANWESHA
ANWITA
ANWYN
ANXHELA
ANYA

ANYA-ROSE
ANYAH
ANYSHA
ANYSIA
ANYSSA
ANZA
ANZAL
ANZAR
ANZILA
AODAN
AODHAN
AOIBH
AOIBHE
AOIBHEANN
AOIBHIN
AOIBHINN
AOIFE
AOIFE-BELLE
AOIFE-ROSE
AOIFFE
AOKI
AOLANI
AOUN
AOUS
APARNA
APHIA
APHINA
APHRA
APHRODITE
APISAN
APISHA
APOLLINE
APOLLO
APOLLON
APOLLONIA
APOLONIA
APPHIA
APPLE
APRIL
APRIL-LOUISE
APRIL-ROSE
APRYL
APSARA
AQEEB
AQEEL
AQEELA
AQEELAH
AQEIL

AQIB
AQIL
AQILA
AQILAH
AQSA
AQSAA
AQSAH
AQUA
AQUEELAH
AQUIB
AQUILA
ARA
ARABA
ARABEL
ARABELLA
ARABELLA-GRACE
ARABELLA-ROSE
ARABELLE
ARAD
ARADHANA
ARADHYA
ARAF
ARAFA
ARAFAAT
ARAFAH
ARAFAT
ARAFATH
ARAGORN
ARAIYA
ARAIZ
ARALIYA
ARAM
ARAMIDE
ARAMINTA
ARAMIS
ARAN
ARANDEEP
ARANDIP
ARANI
ARANJIT
ARANN
ARANTXA
ARANVEER
ARAOLUWA
ARAS
ARASH
ARATI
ARAV
ARAVIND
ARAYA
ARAYAH
ARAYAN
ARAZ
ARBA
ARBAAZ
ARBAB
ARBAS
ARBAZ
ARBELLA
ARBEN
ARBER
ARBESA
ARBI
ARBIE
ARBNOR
ARBRI
ARBY
ARCHANA
ARCHEE
ARCHER
ARCHEY
ARCHI
ARCHIBALD
ARCHIBOLD
ARCHIE
ARCHIE-GEORGE
ARCHIE-J
ARCHIE-JACK
ARCHIE-JAI
ARCHIE-JAMES
ARCHIE-JAY
ARCHIE-JOE
ARCHIE-JOHN
ARCHIE-LEE
ARCHIE-LEIGH
ARCHIE-RAY
ARCHIEBALD
ARCHIMEDES
ARCHISHA
ARCHIT
ARCHITA
ARCHNA
ARCHY
ARDA
ARDAN
ARDEN
ARDI
ARDIAN
ARDIL
ARDIT
ARDITA
AREEB
AREEBA
AREEBAH
AREECE
AREEF
AREEFA
AREEHA
AREEJ
AREEN
AREENA
AREES
AREESA
AREESHA
AREEZ
AREEZA
AREFA
AREL
ARELLA
AREN
ARENA
ARES
ARESHA
ARETAS
ARETHA
ARETI
AREYA
AREZ
ARFA
ARFAH
ARFAN
ARFATH
ARFON
ARGJENT
ARHAA
ARHAAM
ARHAAN
ARHAM
ARHAN
ARHUM
ARI
ARIA
ARIA-JANE
ARIA-MAE

ARIA-MAY	ARIJA	ARKAN
ARIA-RAE	ARIJIELE	ARKIN
ARIA-ROSE	ARIJUS	ARLA
ARIAANA	ARIK	ARLA-RAE
ARIADNA	ARIKA	ARLA-ROSE
ARIADNE	ARIN	ARLAN
ARIADNI	ARINA	ARLANDRIA
ARIAH	ARINI	ARLEIGH
ARIAL	ARINOLA	ARLEN
ARIAM	ARINZE	ARLENE
ARIAN	ARINZECHUKWU	ARLETTE
ARIANA	ARIO	ARLEY
ARIANA-ROSE	ARIOLA	ARLEYA
ARIANAH	ARION	ARLI
ARIANE	ARIONA	ARLIA
ARIANNA	ARIOS	ARLIE
ARIANNA-ROSE	ARIQ	ARLIND
ARIANNAH	ARIS	ARLINDA
ARIANNE	ARISA	ARLO
ARIANWEN	ARISH	ARLO-JAMES
ARIARNA	ARISHA	ARLO-JAY
ARIAS	ARISSA	ARLOH
ARIB	ARISTOTELIS	ARLOW
ARIBA	ARITA	ARLOWE
ARIBAH	ARIUS	ARMAAN
ARIBELLA	ARIV	ARMAANI
ARIC	ARIYA	ARMAN
ARIE	ARIYAAN	ARMAND
ARIEL	ARIYAH	ARMANDA
ARIELA	ARIYAH-ROSE	ARMANDAS
ARIELE	ARIYAN	ARMANDEEP
ARIELLA	ARIYANA	ARMANDO
ARIELLE	ARIYANNA	ARMANDS
ARIEN	ARIYO	ARMANI
ARIENNA	ARIZ	ARMANIE
ARIENNE	ARIZONA	ARMANJ
ARIETA	ARJAN	ARMANN
ARIETTA	ARJAY	ARMARI
ARIF	ARJEN	ARMARNI
ARIFA	ARJIN	ARMEEN
ARIFAH	ARJON	ARMEL
ARIFUL	ARJUN	ARMELA
ARIFUR	ARJUNA	ARMELLE
ARIHAAN	ARJUNAN	ARMEN
ARIHAN	ARJUNVEER	ARMEND
ARIHANNA	ARKA	ARMIN
ARIHANT	ARKADIUSZ	ARMINA
ARIJ	ARKADY	ARMINAS

ARMITA
ARMON
ARNA
ARNALDO
ARNAS
ARNAUD
ARNAV
ARNE
ARNELA
ARNEZ
ARNI
ARNICA
ARNIE
ARNIKA
ARNIS
ARNISA
ARNIT
ARNO
ARNOLD
ARNOLDAS
ARNYA
ARO
AROHA
AROHI
AROLD
ARON
ARONAS
ARONDEEP
AROOB
AROOBA
AROOJ
AROON
AROOSA
AROOSH
AROOSHA
ARORA
AROS
AROUGE
AROUSA
AROUSH
AROZ
ARPAD
ARPAN
ARPIT
ARPITA
ARQAM
ARRABELLA
ARRAN

ARREN
ARRIA
ARRIANA
ARRIANNA
ARRIANNE
ARRIE
ARRIELLA
ARRIETTY
ARRISON
ARRON
ARRON-JUNIOR
ARRUN
ARRY
ARSAL
ARSALAAN
ARSALAN
ARSEMA
ARSEN
ARSENE
ARSENIJ
ARSENIY
ARSH
ARSHA
ARSHAAN
ARSHAD
ARSHAN
ARSHDEEP
ARSHEEN
ARSHI
ARSHIA
ARSHIDA
ARSHIN
ARSHIYA
ARSHMAN
ARSHPREET
ARSHVEER
ARSLAAN
ARSLAN
ART
ARTA
ARTAN
ARTE
ARTEM
ARTEMAS
ARTEMIJS
ARTEMIS
ARTEMISIA
ARTEMIY

ARTEMUS
ARTEMY
ARTH
ARTHAV
ARTHI
ARTHUR
ARTHUR-GEORGE
ARTHUR-JAMES
ARTHUR-JOHN
ARTI
ARTIE
ARTIN
ARTINA
ARTIOLA
ARTIOM
ARTIS
ARTJOM
ARTJOMS
ARTO
ARTUR
ARTURAS
ARTURO
ARTURS
ARTY
ARTYOM
ARUB
ARUBA
ARUBAH
ARUJ
ARUJAN
ARUL
ARUN
ARUNA
ARUNAS
ARUNDEEP
ARUNJIT
ARUNVEER
ARUNVIR
ARUSA
ARUSH
ARUSHA
ARUSHAN
ARUSHI
ARVAN
ARVEEN
ARVI
ARVID
ARVIN

ARVIND	ASEDA	ASHFORD
ARVINDER	ASEEB	ASHI
ARWA	ASEEL	ASHIA
ARWAA	ASEEM	ASHIK
ARWAH	ASEES	ASHIKA
ARWAND	ASEL	ASHIL
ARWEL	ASEN	ASHIM
ARWEN	ASENA	ASHIR
ARWENNA	ASENAT	ASHIRA
ARWIN	ASENATH	ASHISH
ARWYN	ASER	ASHITA
ARYA	ASEYA	ASHIYA
ARYAA	ASFA	ASHKAN
ARYAAN	ASFIYA	ASHLAN
ARYAHI	ASGER	ASHLEA
ARYAM	ASGHAR	ASHLEAH
ARYAMAN	ASH	ASHLEE
ARYAN	ASH-LEIGH	ASHLEEN
ARYANA	ASHA	ASHLEI
ARYANNA	ASHAAN	ASHLEIGH
ARYAV	ASHAI	ASHLEIGH-ANN
ARYAVEER	ASHAL	ASHLEIGH-ANNE
ARYAZ	ASHALINA	ASHLEIGH-JADE
ARYE	ASHAN	ASHLEIGH-LOUISE
ARYEH	ASHANA	ASHLEIGH-MARIE
ARYIA	ASHANI	ASHLEIGH-MAY
ARYN	ASHANTA	ASHLEIGH-PAIGE
ARYO	ASHANTAE	ASHLEIGH-ROSE
ARZAAN	ASHANTAY	ASHLEY
ARZHIN	ASHANTE	ASHLEY-JAMES
ARZO	ASHANTI	ASHLEY-JUNIOR
ARZOO	ASHANTI-LEIGH	ASHLEYNE
ARZU	ASHANTIA	ASHLI
AS'AD	ASHAR	ASHLIE
ASA	ASHARN	ASHLIEGH
ASAAD	ASHARNA	ASHLIN
ASAD	ASHAY	ASHLING
ASADULLAH	ASHAYA	ASHLY
ASAF	ASHAYLA	ASHLYN
ASAIAH	ASHAZ	ASHLYNN
ASAL	ASHBIE	ASHLYNNE
ASAM	ASHBY	ASHMAAN
ASAN	ASHDEEP	ASHMEEN
ASANTE	ASHDEN	ASHMEET
ASAPH	ASHDON	ASHMI
ASAR	ASHEKA	ASHMIT
ASARU	ASHER	ASHMITA
ASBAH	ASHFAQ	ASHMITHA

ASHNA	ASIYA	ASTOR
ASHNI	ASIYAH	ASTRA
ASHOK	ASIYE	ASTRID
ASHON	ASJAD	ASTYN
ASHPREET	ASLAM	ASUKA
ASHRAF	ASLAN	ASVIN
ASHRAFUL	ASLI	ASWIN
ASHRIEL	ASMA	ASWINI
ASHTEN	ASMAA	ASYA
ASHTON	ASMAH	ATA
ASHTON-JAMES	ASMARA	ATAKAN
ASHTON-JAY	ASMI	ATAL
ASHTON-LEE	ASMIN	ATALANTA
ASHTON-THOMAS	ASMITA	ATALIA
ASHTYN	ASMITHA	ATALIAH
ASHUR	ASNA	ATALYA
ASHVATH	ASPEN	ATANAS
ASHVEEN	ASRA	ATARA
ASHVEER	ASRAA	ATARAH
ASHVI	ASRAF	ATAS
ASHVIK	ASRIEL	ATEEB
ASHVIKA	ASSAD	ATEEQ
ASHVIN	ASSAM	ATEEQA
ASHVINA	ASSAN	ATEEYAH
ASHVINI	ASSEM	ATENA
ASHVIR	ASSER	ATENE
ASHWAQ	ASSIA	ATES
ASHWATH	ASSIATOU	ATHALIA
ASHWIKA	ASSIM	ATHALIE
ASHWIN	ASSISI	ATHAN
ASHWINA	ASSIYA	ATHANASIA
ASHWINI	ASSIYAH	ATHANASIOS
ASHWYN	ASSMA	ATHAR
ASIA	ASSUMPTA	ATHARV
ASIA'H	ASSUNTA	ATHARVA
ASIAH	ASTA	ATHAVAN
ASID	ASTALA	ATHEA
ASIER	ASTARA	ATHELSTAN
ASIF	ASTEN	ATHENA
ASIFA	ASTER	ATHENA-ROSE
ASIL	ASTERA	ATHENE
ASILA	ASTHA	ATHINA
ASILAH	ASTIJUS	ATHIRA
ASIM	ASTIN	ATHIYA
ASIMA	ASTON	ATHOS
ASIMINA	ASTON-JAMES	ATHUL
ASIN	ASTON-JAY	ATHULYA
ASIR	ASTON-LEE	ATIA

ATIAH	AUDREY	AURYN
ATIF	AUDRIE	AUSAR
ATIFA	AUDRINA	AUSTEJA
ATIFAH	AUGUST	AUSTEN
ATIKA	AUGUSTA	AUSTIN
ATIKAH	AUGUSTAS	AUSTIN-JAMES
ATIKSH	AUGUSTE	AUSTINE
ATILA	AUGUSTIN	AUSTYN
ATILLA	AUGUSTINA	AUTUM
ATINA	AUGUSTINAS	AUTUMN
ATINUKE	AUGUSTINE	AUTUMN-GRACE
ATIQ	AUGUSTO	AUTUMN-LILY
ATIQA	AUGUSTUS	AUTUMN-ROSE
ATISH	AUKSE	AUTUMN-WILLOW
ATIYA	AULON	AUZAIR
ATIYAH	AULONA	AVA
ATIYYA	AUM	AVA-
ATIYYAH	AUN	AVA-ANN
ATLANTA	AURA	AVA-BELLE
ATLANTIS	AURALIA	AVA-BLU
ATLAS	AURAYA	AVA-ELIZABETH
ATLEY	AUREA	AVA-FAITH
ATO	AUREJA	AVA-GRACE
ATQIYA	AUREL	AVA-JADE
ATREYU	AURELA	AVA-JAI
ATRINA	AURELIA	AVA-JANE
ATSUSHI	AURELIAN	AVA-JAY
ATTA	AURELIE	AVA-JAYNE
ATTIA	AURELIEN	AVA-JEAN
ATTICA	AURELIJA	AVA-JO
ATTICUS	AURELIO	AVA-LEA
ATTIF	AURELIUS	AVA-LEE
ATTILA	AURI	AVA-LEI
ATTIYA	AURIA	AVA-LEIGH
ATUL	AURIANNA	AVA-LILLIE
AUBERON	AURIEL	AVA-LILLY
AUBIN	AURIELLA	AVA-LILY
AUBREE	AURIKA	AVA-LOUISE
AUBREE-ROSE	AURIOL	AVA-MAE
AUBREY	AURLA	AVA-MAI
AUBREY-ROSE	AURON	AVA-MARIA
AUBRIE	AURORA	AVA-MARIE
AUDE	AURORA-GRACE	AVA-MAY
AUDEN	AURORA-JANE	AVA-NICOLE
AUDIE	AURORA-LEIGH	AVA-RAE
AUDLEY	AURORA-MAE	AVA-RAI
AUDRA	AURORA-MAY	AVA-ROSE
AUDREE	AURORA-ROSE	AVA-RUBY

AVA-SKYE
AVA-SOPHIA
AVA-VIOLET
AVAANA
AVAANI
AVAH
AVAH-ROSE
AVAIAH
AVAIS
AVAIYA
AVAIYAH
AVALEE
AVALEIGH
AVALINE
AVALON
AVALYN
AVALYNN
AVAN
AVANA
AVANEESH
AVANGELINE
AVANI
AVANISH
AVANNA
AVANNAH
AVANTHIKA
AVANTIKA
AVAR
AVARNI
AVAROSE
AVARY
AVAYA
AVAYAH
AVEAH
AVEEN
AVEER
AVELINA
AVELINE
AVELYN
AVEN
AVENA
AVERIE
AVERIL
AVERY
AVESTA
AVEY
AVEYA
AVEYAH

AVI
AVIA
AVIAH
AVIANA
AVIANNA
AVIARNA
AVIDAN
AVIE
AVIEL
AVIELA
AVIELLA
AVIGAIL
AVIGAYIL
AVIGDOR
AVIGHNA
AVIJOT
AVIK
AVIKA
AVIN
AVINA
AVINAASH
AVINASH
AVIR
AVIRAJ
AVIRAL
AVISH
AVISHA
AVISHAI
AVISHI
AVITA
AVITAL
AVIV
AVIVA
AVIYA
AVLEEN
AVNEE
AVNEET
AVNER
AVNI
AVNISH
AVNOOR
AVRAHAM
AVRAJ
AVRAM
AVREET
AVRIL
AVROHAM
AVROHOM

AVRUM
AVRUMI
AVTAR
AVY
AVYA
AVYAAN
AVYAN
AVYANNA
AVYUKT
AVYUKTH
AWA
AWAAB
AWAB
AWAD
AWAIS
AWAIZ
AWATIF
AWEL
AWEN
AWENA
AWESOME
AWIN
AWO
AWS
AWSTIN
AWURA
AWWAB
AWWAL
AXEL
AXELLE
AXL
AXTON
AYA
AYAA
AYAAH
AYAAN
AYAANA
AYAANAH
AYAANSH
AYAAT
AYAAZ
AYAD
AYAH
AYAH-NOOR
AYAKA
AYALA
AYAN
AYANA

AYANAH	AYLA-LOUISE	AYRAH
AYANDA	AYLA-MAE	AYRAN
AYANE	AYLA-MAI	AYRON
AYANFEOLUWA	AYLA-MAY	AYRTON
AYANLE	AYLA-RAE	AYSA
AYANNA	AYLA-ROSE	AYSE
AYANNAH	AYLAH	AYSEGUL
AYANO	AYLAN	AYSEL
AYANSH	AYLAR	AYSEM
AYASHA	AYLEEN	AYSENUR
AYAT	AYLESHA	AYSER
AYATH	AYLIN	AYSHA
AYAZ	AYLINE	AYSHAH
AYCA	AYLISH	AYSHE
AYCAN	AYLISHA	AYSHEA
AYCE	AYMA	AYSHIA
AYDA	AYMAAN	AYSIA
AYDA-GRACE	AYMAN	AYSU
AYDA-ROSE	AYMARA	AYTEN
AYDAN	AYMEE	AYUB
AYDEN	AYMEN	AYUMI
AYDENN	AYMERIC	AYUSH
AYDIN	AYMIE	AYUSHI
AYDN	AYMIRA	AYUSHMA
AYDON	AYNA	AYUUB
AYE	AYNI	AYVA
AYEASHA	AYNSLEY	AYVA-MAE
AYEESHA	AYNUR	AYVA-ROSE
AYEISHA	AYO	AYVAH
AYELA	AYOBAMI	AYYAAN
AYELET	AYODEJI	AYYAN
AYESH	AYODELE	AYYASH
AYESHA	AYOKUNLE	AYYAT
AYESHAH	AYOKUNMI	AYYOUB
AYESHIA	AYOMIDE	AYYUB
AYET	AYOMIKUN	AYZA
AYEZA	AYOMIPO	AYZAH
AYHAM	AYOMIPOSI	AZAAN
AYHAN	AYON	AZAD
AYHEM	AYONA	AZAELIA
AYIA	AYONITEMI	AZAHLIA
AYIANA	AYOOB	AZAI
AYISHA	AYOOLA	AZAIAH
AYISHAH	AYOOLUWA	AZAL
AYKUT	AYOTOMIWA	AZALEA
AYLA	AYOTUNDE	AZALIA
AYLA-GRACE	AYOUB	AZALIAH
AYLA-JADE	AYRA	AZAM

AZAN
AZANIA
AZAR
AZARA
AZARI
AZARIA
AZARIAH
AZAT
AZAYAH
AZBAH
AZEALIA
AZEEM
AZEEMA
AZEEMAH
AZEEN
AZEEZ
AZEEZA
AZEEZAH
AZEEZAT
AZEL
AZFAR
AZHAAN
AZHAAR
AZHAR
AZHARUL
AZIA
AZIAH
AZIB
AZIEL
AZIL
AZIM
AZIMA
AZITA
AZIYAH
AZIZ
AZIZA
AZIZAH
AZIZE
AZIZUL
AZIZUR
AZKA
AZLAAN
AZLAN
AZMA
AZMAT
AZMEENA
AZMEER
AZMINA

AZRA
AZRAA
AZRAEL
AZRAF
AZRAH
AZRIEL
AZUOLAS
AZURA
AZWA
AZYAN
AZZA
AZZAH
AZZAM
AZZURRA

B

B'ELANNA
BAABA
BAANI
BAASIT
BABA
BABAFEMI
BABAJIDE
BABAK
BABAN
BABAR
BABATUNDE
BABER
BABETTE
BABITA
BABOUCARR
BABUCARR
BABY
BADAL
BADAR
BADE
BADEN
BADER
BADR
BADRIYA
BAE
BAFFOUR
BAHADAR
BAHAND
BAHAR
BAHARA
BAHEER
BAHEZ
BAHISHT
BAHJA
BAHOZ
BAHRAM
BAI
BAIDEN
BAILA
BAILEA
BAILEE
BAILEIGH
BAILEY
BAILEY-ANNE

BAILEY-GRACE
BAILEY-JAMES
BAILEY-JAY
BAILEY-JOE
BAILEY-LEE
BAILEY-MAE
BAILEY-MAI
BAILEY-MAY
BAILEY-RAE
BAILEY-RAY
BAILEY-ROSE
BAILIE
BAILIN
BAILLIE
BAILY
BAINE
BAKARI
BAKARY
BAKER
BAKHTAWAR
BAKHTIYAR
BAKIR
BAKO
BAKR
BALAAL
BALAJI
BALAL
BALAZS
BALBIR
BALDEEP
BALDWIN
BALE
BALEN
BALI
BALIAN
BALIN
BALINT
BALJEET
BALJINDER
BALJIT
BALJOT
BALLAL
BALPREET
BALQEES
BALQIS
BALRAJ
BALRAM
BALROOP

BALSAM
BALTAZAR
BALTEJ
BALTHAZAR
BALVEER
BAM
BAMBI
BAMIDELE
BANA
BANAN
BANE
BANEEN
BANEET
BANI
BANITA
BANSARI
BANSI
BANSRI
BANU
BANUJAN
BAO
BAPTISTE
BAQIR
BARAA
BARACK
BARAKA
BARAKAH
BARAKAT
BARAN
BARBARA
BARBOD
BARBORA
BARCLAY
BARCLEY
BARDIA
BAREEHA
BAREEN
BAREERA
BAREERAH
BAREZ
BARIMA
BARIN
BARIRA
BARIRAH
BARIS
BARKLEY
BARLEY
BARNABAS

BARNABY
BARNES
BARNEY
BARNI
BARNIE
BARNY
BARON
BARRIE
BARRINGTON
BARRY
BARSAM
BART
BARTEK
BARTHOLOMEW
BARTLOMIEJ
BARTON
BARTOSZ
BARUCH
BARUN
BARZAN
BASAK
BASEL
BASEM
BASHAR
BASHEER
BASHIR
BASIL
BASILE
BASIM
BASIR
BASIT
BASMA
BASMAH
BASMALA
BASRA
BASSAM
BASSEL
BASSI
BASSIM
BASSY
BASTIAN
BASTIEN
BASYA
BATHSHEBA
BATOOL
BATOUL
BATSHEVA
BATU

BATUHAN
BATUL
BATYA
BAVISHA
BAVITA
BAVLEEN
BAVNEET
BAWAN
BAWAR
BAWER
BAXTER
BAY
BAYA
BAYAAN
BAYAN
BAYDEN
BAYE
BAYLA
BAYLEA
BAYLEE
BAYLEIGH
BAYLEIGH-MAE
BAYLEN
BAYLEY
BAYLIE
BAYRAM
BAZIL
BEA
BEAR
BEATA
BEATRICE
BEATRIS
BEATRISA
BEATRISE
BEATRIX
BEATRIZ
BEATTIE
BEAU
BEAU-LILY
BEAUDEN
BEAUMONT
BEAUREGARD
BEAUTY
BEAUX
BEBE
BECA
BECCA
BECCI

BECK
BECKETT
BECKHAM
BECKI
BECKIE
BECKS
BECKY
BEDE
BEDIRHAN
BEDRAN
BEDWYR
BEE
BEENISH
BEGUM
BEGW
BEHESHTA
BEHRAM
BEHROUZ
BEHZAD
BEIBHINN
BEILA
BEILY
BEJNA
BEKI
BEKIM
BEKIR
BEKKI
BELA
BELAL
BELEN
BELICIA
BELIEVE
BELINA
BELINAY
BELINDA
BELIS
BELLA
BELLA-
BELLA-ANN
BELLA-BEAU
BELLA-GRACE
BELLA-IVY
BELLA-JADE
BELLA-LOUISE
BELLA-MAE
BELLA-MAI
BELLA-MARIA
BELLA-MARIE

BELLA-MAY
BELLA-MIA
BELLA-RAE
BELLA-RENEE
BELLA-ROSE
BELLAMY
BELLANGE
BELLAROSE
BELLATRIX
BELLE
BELTRAN
BELYNDA
BEN
BENAIAH
BENARD
BENAS
BENAZIR
BENCE
BENDE
BENDEGUZ
BENEAMIN
BENEDEK
BENEDETTA
BENEDICT
BENEDICTA
BENEDICTE
BENEDIKT
BENEDIKTAS
BENET
BENETT
BENHUR
BENI
BENIAH
BENIAMIN
BENICIA
BENICIO
BENIN
BENITA
BENITO
BENJAMAN
BENJAMEN
BENJAMIM
BENJAMIN
BENJAMIN-JAMES
BENJAMINE
BENJAMYN
BENJI
BENJIMAN

BENJIMIN
BENJY
BENN
BENNET
BENNETT
BENNI
BENNIE
BENNY
BENOIT
BENSON
BENTE
BENTLEE
BENTLEY
BENTLY
BENTON
BENYAMEEN
BENYAMIN
BENZION
BERAN
BERAT
BERAY
BERCEM
BERDAN
BEREKET
BEREN
BERENICE
BERENIKA
BERES
BERFIN
BERHAN
BERI
BERIL
BERIN
BERISH
BERITAN
BERIVAN
BERK
BERKAN
BERKAY
BERKE
BERKIN
BERNA
BERNADETTE
BERNADINE
BERNARD
BERNARDAS
BERNARDO
BERNICE

BERNIE
BERRA
BERRI
BERRIE
BERRIN
BERRY
BERT
BERTA
BERTAN
BERTHA
BERTIE
BERTRAM
BERTRAND
BERTY
BERYL
BERZAN
BESARTA
BESIAN
BESIANA
BESMIR
BESNIK
BESS
BESSIE
BESSY
BESTE
BETANIA
BETH
BETH-ANNE
BETHAN
BETHANE
BETHANEE
BETHANEY
BETHANI
BETHANIE
BETHANN
BETHANNEY
BETHANNIE
BETHANY
BETHANY-
BETHANY-ANN
BETHANY-ANNE
BETHANY-JADE
BETHANY-JANE
BETHANY-JAYNE
BETHANY-JO
BETHANY-LOUISE
BETHANY-MAE
BETHANY-MAI

BETHANY-MARIE	BEXLEY	BIJAL
BETHANY-MAY	BEYLA	BIJAN
BETHANY-PAIGE	BEYONCE	BIJOU
BETHANY-ROSE	BEYZA	BIKRAM
BETHEL	BEYZANUR	BIKRAMJIT
BETHEN	BEZALEL	BILAAL
BETHENY	BEZAWIT	BILAL
BETHIA	BHADRA	BILAN
BETHINN	BHAIRAVI	BILAWAL
BETHLEHEM	BHAKTI	BILGE
BETHNEY	BHARAT	BILL
BETHONY	BHARATH	BILLAL
BETI	BHARGAV	BILLI
BETIEL	BHARGAVI	BILLI-JO
BETIM	BHAVAN	BILLIE
BETSAN	BHAVANA	BILLIE-
BETSEY	BHAVANDEEP	BILLIE-ANN
BETSI	BHAVDEEP	BILLIE-ANNE
BETSIE	BHAVEN	BILLIE-JADE
BETSIE-MAE	BHAVESH	BILLIE-JANE
BETSY	BHAVI	BILLIE-JAY
BETSY-BLU	BHAVIK	BILLIE-JEAN
BETSY-BO	BHAVIKA	BILLIE-JO
BETSY-LOU	BHAVIN	BILLIE-JOE
BETSY-MAE	BHAVINA	BILLIE-LEA
BETSY-MAY	BHAVINI	BILLIE-LEIGH
BETSY-RAE	BHAVISH	BILLIE-LOUISE
BETSY-ROSE	BHAVISHA	BILLIE-MAE
BETTE	BHAVISHYA	BILLIE-MAI
BETTIE	BHAVJOT	BILLIE-MARIE
BETTINA	BHAVNA	BILLIE-MAY
BETTSIE	BHAVNEET	BILLIE-RAE
BETTSY	BHAVYA	BILLIE-ROSE
BETTY	BHOOMI	BILLIEJO
BETTY-LOU	BHUMI	BILLY
BETTY-MAE	BHUMIKA	BILLY-DEAN
BETTY-MAY	BHUPINDER	BILLY-GEORGE
BETTY-ROSE	BHUVAN	BILLY-JAMES
BETUEL	BHUVI	BILLY-JAY
BETUL	BIA	BILLY-JO
BETZALEL	BIAGIO	BILLY-JOE
BEULAH	BIANCA	BILLY-JOHN
BEVAN	BIANCA-MARIA	BILLY-LEE
BEVERLEY	BIANKA	BILLY-RAE
BEVERLY	BIBA	BILLY-RAY
BEVIN	BIBI	BILLY-THOMAS
BEVIS	BIBIANA	BILLYBOB
BEVON	BIDDY	BILLYJOE

BILLYLEE	BLAYDEN	BOBBI-LEIGH
BILLYRAY	BLAYKE	BOBBI-LOU
BILQEES	BLAYN	BOBBI-MAE
BILQIS	BLAYNE	BOBBI-MARIE
BINA	BLAYZE	BOBBI-ROSE
BINAL	BLAZE	BOBBIE
BINDI	BLAZEJ	BOBBIE-ANN
BING	BLEDDYN	BOBBIE-JADE
BINIAM	BLEN	BOBBIE-JO
BINKY	BLEND	BOBBIE-LEE
BINTA	BLENDA	BOBBIE-LEIGH
BINTOU	BLENDI	BOBBIE-MAE
BINTU	BLEON	BOBBIE-MAY
BINYAMEEN	BLEONA	BOBBIE-RAE
BINYAMIN	BLERIM	BOBBIE-ROSE
BINYOMIN	BLERINA	BOBBY
BIPASHA	BLERON	BOBBY-DEAN
BIRDIE	BLERTA	BOBBY-GEORGE
BIRRAH	BLERTON	BOBBY-JACK
BISHAN	BLESS	BOBBY-JAI
BISHOP	BLESSED	BOBBY-JAMES
BISMA	BLESSING	BOBBY-JAY
BISMAH	BLESSINGS	BOBBY-JO
BISOLA	BLEU	BOBBY-JOE
BITA	BLIMA	BOBBY-JOHN
BITANIA	BLIMI	BOBBY-LEE
BIVON	BLIN	BOBBY-PAUL
BJORN	BLINA	BOBBY-RAY
BLADE	BLISS	BOBBYJOE
BLADEN	BLOSSOM	BOBI
BLAIDD	BLOUSEY	BODE
BLAIKE	BLOUSIE	BODEN
BLAIN	BLU	BODHI
BLAINE	BLU-BELLE	BODI
BLAIR	BLUBELLE	BODIE
BLAIRE	BLUE	BODRUL
BLAISE	BLUEBELL	BOE
BLAITHIN	BLUEBELLE	BOGDAN
BLAIZE	BLYSS	BOGLARKA
BLAKE	BLYTH	BOGOMIL
BLAKELEY	BLYTHE	BOHAN
BLAKELY	BO	BOHDAN
BLANAID	BOADICEA	BOHDI
BLANCA	BOAZ	BOHEN
BLANCHE	BOB	BOJIDAR
BLANE	BOBBI	BOLUWATIFE
BLANKA	BOBBI-JO	BON
BLAYDE	BOBBI-LEE	BONHAM

BONIFACE	BOZENA	BRANDO
BONITA	BOZHIDAR	BRANDON
BONNEE	BOZHIDARA	BRANDON-
BONNI	BRACHA	BRANDON-JAMES
BONNIE	BRACKEN	BRANDON-LEE
BONNIE-BLU	BRAD	BRANDON-LEIGH
BONNIE-BLUE	BRAD-LEE	BRANDONLEE
BONNIE-LEE	BRADAN	BRANDY
BONNIE-LEIGH	BRADD	BRANDYN
BONNIE-LOU	BRADEN	BRANNAGH
BONNIE-LOUISE	BRADEY	BRANNAN
BONNIE-MAE	BRADIE	BRANNON
BONNIE-MAI	BRADLEE	BRANON
BONNIE-MARIE	BRADLEIGH	BRANSON
BONNIE-MAY	BRADLEY	BRANT
BONNIE-RAE	BRADLEY-JAMES	BRANWEN
BONNIE-ROSE	BRADLEY-JOHN	BRAULIO
BONNY	BRADLIE	BRAX
BONO	BRADLY	BRAXSON
BOO	BRADON	BRAXSTON
BOOKER	BRADY	BRAXTON
BORA	BRADYN	BRAY
BORAN	BRAE	BRAYAN
BORBALA	BRAEDAN	BRAYDAN
BORIL	BRAEDEN	BRAYDEN
BORIS	BRAEDON	BRAYDEN-LEE
BORISLAV	BRAEDYN	BRAYDN
BORUCH	BRAELYN	BRAYDON
BORYS	BRAHIM	BRAYEN
BOSCO	BRAIAN	BRAYLAN
BOSHRA	BRAIDAN	BRAYLEIGH
BOSTON	BRAIDEN	BRAYLEN
BOTAN	BRAIDEN-LEE	BRAYLIN
BOTOND	BRAIDON	BRAYLON
BOUBACAR	BRAIDY	BRAYSON
BOUCHRA	BRAIENS	BREA
BOUDICA	BRAITH	BREAGH
BOUDICCA	BRAJAN	BREAGHA
BOUX	BRAJEN	BREAH
BOW	BRAM	BREANA
BOWDEN	BRAMLEY	BREANNA
BOWE	BRAMWELL	BREANNE
BOWEN	BRAN	BRECCAN
BOWIE	BRANDAN	BRECKIN
BOYAN	BRANDEN	BRECON
BOYCE	BRANDEN-LEE	BREDA
BOYCIE	BRANDI	BREE
BOYD	BRANDIE	BREEANNA

BREEYA
BREEZE
BREINDEL
BREINDY
BREMNER
BREN
BRENDA
BRENDAN
BRENDAN-LEE
BRENDEN
BRENDON
BRENDYN
BRENIN
BRENNA
BRENNAN
BRENNEN
BRENNIG
BRENNON
BRENT
BRENTLEY
BRENTON
BRESHNA
BRET
BRETT
BRETTON
BREYA
BREYANA
BREYANNA
BREYDON
BRIA
BRIALLEN
BRIAN
BRIANA
BRIANIE
BRIANNA
BRIANNA-LEIGH
BRIANNAH
BRIANNE
BRIANNY
BRIANY
BRIAR
BRIAR-ROSE
BRIARNA
BRICE
BRIDE
BRIDEY
BRIDGET
BRIDGETTE

BRIDGIE
BRIDIE
BRIDIE-LEIGH
BRIE
BRIEANNA
BRIEGE
BRIELLA
BRIELLE
BRIENNE
BRIER
BRIERLEY
BRIGHT
BRIGID
BRIGIT
BRIGITA
BRIGITTE
BRIHANNA
BRIJESH
BRILEY
BRIN
BRINDA
BRINDLEY
BRINLEY
BRIONEY
BRIONI
BRIONIE
BRIONNY
BRIONY
BRISEIS
BRISHNA
BRISHTI
BRITANEY
BRITANI
BRITANIA
BRITANIE
BRITANNI
BRITANNIA
BRITANNY
BRITANY
BRITENY
BRITHANY
BRITNEE
BRITNEY
BRITNIE
BRITTANEY
BRITTANI
BRITTANIE
BRITTANNY

BRITTANY
BRITTENY
BRITTNEY
BRITTONY
BRIXTON
BRIYANA
BROC
BROCHA
BROCHO
BROCK
BRODAN
BRODEE
BRODEN
BRODERICK
BRODEY
BRODHI
BRODI
BRODIE
BRODIE-LEE
BRODIE-LEIGH
BRODY
BRODY-LEE
BROGAN
BROGAN-LEE
BROGEN
BROGHAN
BROGUN
BROMLEY
BROMWYN
BRONAGH
BRONIA
BRONNEN
BRONSON
BRONTE
BRONTI
BRONTIE
BRONTY
BRONWEN
BRONWYN
BRONYA
BROOK
BROOKE
BROOKE-AMELIA
BROOKE-ELISE
BROOKE-LEA
BROOKE-LEIGH
BROOKE-LOUISE
BROOKE-LYN

BROOKE-LYNN
BROOKE-MARIE
BROOKE-ROSE
BROOKELYN
BROOKLAN
BROOKLIN
BROOKLYN
BROOKLYN-LEE
BROOKLYN-MAI
BROOKLYN-ROSE
BROOKLYNE
BROOKLYNN
BROOKLYNNE
BROOKS
BRUCE
BRUCHA
BRUCHI
BRUIN
BRUK
BRUNA
BRUNELLA
BRUNO
BRUNON
BRUSK
BRYAN
BRYANA
BRYANIE
BRYANNA
BRYANT
BRYANY
BRYCE
BRYCEN
BRYCHAN
BRYDEN
BRYDIE
BRYDON
BRYHER
BRYLEE
BRYLEIGH
BRYLEY
BRYN
BRYNA
BRYNIE
BRYNLEE
BRYNLEY
BRYNMOR
BRYNN
BRYON
BRYONEY
BRYONI
BRYONIE
BRYONNY
BRYONY
BRYSON
BRYTHON
BUBACARR
BUCK
BUCKLEY
BUDDIE
BUDDUG
BUDDY
BUKET
BUKHARI
BULENT
BULUT
BUNNIE
BUNNY
BUNTY
BUNYAMIN
BUPE
BURAK
BURCIN
BURCU
BURHAAN
BURHAN
BURHANUDDIN
BURT
BURTON
BUSBY
BUSE
BUSHRA
BUSHRAA
BUSHRAH
BUSRA
BUSTER
BUTHAYNA
BUZZ
BYRAN
BYREN
BYRON

C

C
C-JAY
CAAN
CABDI
CABHAN
CACEY
CACIA
CACIE
CADAN
CADANCE
CADE
CADEE
CADEL
CADELL
CADEN
CADEN-JAMES
CADEN-LEE
CADENCE
CADEY
CADHLA
CADI
CADI-MAI
CADIE
CADIE-LEIGH
CADON
CADY
CADYN
CAE
CAEDAN
CAEDEN
CAEDMON
CAEDON
CAEDYN
CAEL
CAELA
CAELAB
CAELAN
CAELEB
CAELEN
CAELI
CAELIA
CAELIN
CAELUM
CAELYN
CAEN
CAERA
CAERAN
CAERON
CAERWYN
CAESAR
CAETANO
CAGAN
CAGDAS
CAGLA
CAHAL
CAHILL
CAI
CAIA
CAIAN
CAICEY
CAID
CAIDAN
CAIDE
CAIDEN
CAIDEN-JAMES
CAIDEN-LEE
CAIDENCE
CAIDON
CAIDY
CAILA
CAILAN
CAILEAN
CAILEB
CAILEIGH
CAILEM
CAILEN
CAILEY
CAILIN
CAILLEN
CAILUM
CAILYN
CAIN
CAINAN
CAINE
CAIO
CAIRA
CAIRAN
CAIRO
CAIRON
CAISEY
CAISHA
CAISON
CAIT
CAITHLIN
CAITIE
CAITLAIN
CAITLAN
CAITLAND
CAITLEN
CAITLIN
CAITLIN-JO
CAITLIN-MAE
CAITLIN-MARIE
CAITLIN-ROSE
CAITLINE
CAITLUN
CAITLYN
CAITLYN-ROSE
CAITLYNN
CAITRIN
CAITRIONA
CAIUS
CAIYA
CAJA
CAL
CALAIS
CALAM
CALAN
CALDER
CALE
CALEB
CALEB-JAMES
CALEDON
CALEESI
CALEIGH
CALEM
CALEN
CALEY
CALI
CALI-ROSE
CALIA
CALIANA
CALIB
CALICO
CALIE
CALIN
CALINA
CALISE
CALISSA
CALISTA

CALIX
CALIXTE
CALLA
CALLAGHAN
CALLAM
CALLAN
CALLEIGH
CALLEM
CALLEN
CALLEY
CALLI
CALLIA
CALLIE
CALLIE-MAE
CALLIE-MAI
CALLIE-MAY
CALLIE-RAE
CALLIE-ROSE
CALLIOPE
CALLISTA
CALLIUM
CALLON
CALLULA
CALLUM
CALLUM-JAMES
CALLUM-JAY
CALLUM-JOHN
CALLUMN
CALLUN
CALLY
CALOGERO
CALON
CALUB
CALUM
CALUMN
CALVERT
CALVIN
CALVYN
CALYB
CALYPSO
CAM'RON
CAMARA
CAMARAN
CAMARI
CAMARON
CAMBELL
CAMDEN
CAMELIA
CAMELLIA
CAMEO
CAMERAN
CAMEREN
CAMERON
CAMERON-JAMES
CAMERON-JAY
CAMERON-LEE
CAMERON-LEWIS
CAMI
CAMI-LEIGH
CAMI-LI
CAMILA
CAMILIA
CAMILLA
CAMILLE
CAMILLIA
CAMILO
CAMISHA
CAMMIE
CAMMY
CAMPBELL
CAMRAN
CAMREN
CAMRON
CAMRYN
CAN
CANAAN
CANAN
CANDACE
CANDEECE
CANDELA
CANDI
CANDICE
CANDIDA
CANDIS
CANDISE
CANDY
CANE
CANER
CANSEL
CANSU
CAOIFE
CAOILAINN
CAOILFHINN
CAOILINN
CAOIMHE
CAOIMHIN
CAOL
CAOLAN
CAPRI
CAPRICE
CAPUCINE
CARA
CARA-JANE
CARA-LEIGH
CARA-LOUISE
CARA-MAE
CARA-MAI
CARA-ROSE
CARADOG
CARAGH
CARAH
CARDELL
CAREN
CARENZA
CAREY
CARI
CARI-ANN
CARIAD
CARIANNE
CARICE
CARIDEE
CARIN
CARINA
CARINE
CARINNA
CARIS
CARISMA
CARISS
CARISSA
CARISSE
CARITA
CARL
CARL-JAMES
CARL-JUNIOR
CARLA
CARLA-LOUISE
CARLEE
CARLEIGH
CARLENA
CARLENE
CARLEY
CARLI
CARLIE
CARLIN

CARLISA
CARLISHA
CARLISLE
CARLITA
CARLITO
CARLO
CARLOS
CARLOTA
CARLOTTA
CARLSON
CARLTON
CARLY
CARLY-ANNE
CARLY-JANE
CARLY-RAE
CARLY-ROSE
CARLYLE
CARMA
CARMAN
CARMEL
CARMELA
CARMELITA
CARMELLA
CARMELLE
CARMELO
CARMEN
CARMINA
CARMINE
CARN
CARNELL
CARNEY
CAROL
CAROL-ANN
CAROLA
CAROLANN
CAROLANNE
CAROLE
CAROLINA
CAROLINE
CAROLYN
CAROLYNE
CARON
CARRA
CARRAGH
CARRERA
CARRIANNE
CARRICK
CARRIE

CARRIE-ANN
CARRIE-ANNE
CARRIEANN
CARRIEANNE
CARRIGAN
CARRINA
CARRINGTON
CARRIS
CARSEN
CARSON
CARSON-JAMES
CARSON-LEE
CARSTEN
CARTEL
CARTER
CARTER-JAE
CARTER-JAI
CARTER-JAMES
CARTER-JAY
CARTER-LEE
CARTIER
CARVELL
CARVER
CARWYN
CARY
CARYL
CARYN
CARYS
CAS
CASANDRA
CASE
CASEN
CASEY
CASEY-
CASEY-ANN
CASEY-ANNE
CASEY-JAMES
CASEY-JANE
CASEY-JAY
CASEY-JAYNE
CASEY-JO
CASEY-LEA
CASEY-LEE
CASEY-LEIGH
CASEY-LOUISE
CASEY-MAE
CASEY-MAI
CASEY-MARIE

CASEY-MAY
CASEY-RAE
CASEYLEE
CASEYLEIGH
CASH
CASHEL
CASI
CASIAN
CASIANA
CASIE
CASIE-LEIGH
CASIM
CASIMIR
CASON
CASPAR
CASPER
CASPIAN
CASS
CASSADY
CASSANDRA
CASSEY
CASSI
CASSIA
CASSIAN
CASSIDIE
CASSIDY
CASSIDY-MAE
CASSIDY-ROSE
CASSIE
CASSIE-ANN
CASSIE-LEIGH
CASSIE-MAI
CASSIEL
CASSIEN
CASSIOPEIA
CASSIUS
CASSY
CASTIEL
CASTOR
CASTRO
CATALAYA
CATALEYA
CATALIN
CATALINA
CATARINA
CATE
CATELIN
CATELYN

CATELYNN
CATERINA
CATHAL
CATHAN
CATHARINA
CATHARINE
CATHERINA
CATHERINE
CATHLEEN
CATHRINE
CATHRYN
CATHY
CATIA
CATIE
CATLIN
CATO
CATRIN
CATRINA
CATRIONA
CATRYN
CATTALEYA
CATTLEYA
CAUA
CAULEY
CAVALLI
CAVAN
CAVANI
CAVELL
CAVEN
CAWLEY
CAYA
CAYAN
CAYCE
CAYCEE
CAYCIE
CAYDAN
CAYDE
CAYDEE
CAYDEN
CAYDEN-JAMES
CAYDEN-JAY
CAYDEN-LEE
CAYDENCE
CAYDIE
CAYDN
CAYDON
CAYENNE
CAYLA

CAYLAN
CAYLE
CAYLEB
CAYLEE
CAYLEIGH
CAYLEM
CAYLEN
CAYLEY
CAYLIN
CAYLON
CAYLUM
CAYMAN
CAYNE
CAYO
CAYSIE
CAYSON
CAYTLIN
CE
CEANA
CEANNA
CEARA
CEBRAIL
CECE
CECELIA
CECI
CECIL
CECILE
CECILIA
CECILIE
CECILLE
CECILY
CECYLIA
CEDAR
CEDRI
CEDRIC
CEDRICK
CEE
CEE-JAY
CEEJAY
CEI
CEIAN
CEINWEN
CEIRA
CEIRAN
CEIRE
CEIRION
CEIRON
CEJAY

CELAL
CELENA
CELENE
CELESTE
CELESTIA
CELESTINA
CELESTINE
CELIA
CELIA-ROSE
CELICIA
CELINA
CELINE
CELLAN
CELSEY
CELSIE
CELT
CELTON
CELVIN
CELYN
CEM
CEMAL
CEMALIYE
CEMILE
CEMLYN
CEMRE
CENGIZ
CENGIZHAN
CENK
CENNET
CEPHAS
CEREN
CERI
CERI-ANN
CERI-ANNE
CERIAN
CERIDWEN
CERINE
CERIS
CERISE
CERITH
CERYN
CERYS
CERYS-ANN
CESAR
CESARE
CESCA
CESUR
CET

CETIN
CEYDA
CEYHAN
CEYHUN
CEYLA
CEYLAN
CEYLIN
CEZAR
CEZARA
CEZARY
CHAAYA
CHACE
CHAD
CHADD
CHADLEY
CHADWICK
CHAE
CHAEL
CHAHAT
CHAI
CHAICE
CHAIM
CHAIMA
CHAISE
CHAITANYA
CHAITRA
CHAIYA
CHAKOTAY
CHALICE
CHALLIS
CHAM
CHAMPAGNE
CHAN
CHANA
CHANADE
CHANAE
CHANAH
CHANAI
CHANAIS
CHANAN
CHANAY
CHANAYA
CHANAYE
CHANCE
CHAND
CHANDA
CHANDAN
CHANDANI
CHANDLER
CHANDNI
CHANDON
CHANDRA
CHANDRESH
CHANDRIKA
CHANEL
CHANELL
CHANELLE
CHANG
CHANI
CHANIA
CHANICE
CHANIE
CHANIECE
CHANIEL
CHANIQUE
CHANISE
CHANIYA
CHANNA
CHANNAH
CHANNAY
CHANNEL
CHANNELLE
CHANNING
CHANNON
CHANPREET
CHANSE
CHANTA
CHANTAE
CHANTAI
CHANTAL
CHANTALLE
CHANTAY
CHANTAYA
CHANTE
CHANTEL
CHANTELE
CHANTELL
CHANTELLE
CHANTILLY
CHANYA
CHARA
CHARALAMBOS
CHARAN
CHARBEL
CHARDAE
CHARDAI
CHARDANNAY
CHARDAY
CHARDENAY
CHARDONAI
CHARDONAY
CHARDONEY
CHARDONNAI
CHARDONNAY
CHARELLE
CHARICE
CHARIS
CHARISE
CHARISMA
CHARISSA
CHARISSE
CHARITY
CHARL
CHARLA
CHARLEA
CHARLEE
CHARLEEN
CHARLEIGH
CHARLENE
CHARLES
CHARLES-JUNIOR
CHARLETTE
CHARLEY
CHARLEY-ANN
CHARLEY-ANNE
CHARLEY-JADE
CHARLEY-JO
CHARLEY-LOUISE
CHARLEY-MAE
CHARLEY-MARIE
CHARLEY-MAY
CHARLEY-RAE
CHARLEY-ROSE
CHARLI
CHARLI-ANN
CHARLI-ANNE
CHARLIE
CHARLIE-
CHARLIE-ANN
CHARLIE-ANNE
CHARLIE-CRAIG
CHARLIE-DEAN
CHARLIE-GEORGE
CHARLIE-J

CHARLIE-JACK
CHARLIE-JADE
CHARLIE-JAMES
CHARLIE-JANE
CHARLIE-JAY
CHARLIE-JO
CHARLIE-JOE
CHARLIE-JOHN
CHARLIE-JUNIOR
CHARLIE-LEE
CHARLIE-LEIGH
CHARLIE-LOUISE
CHARLIE-MAE
CHARLIE-MAI
CHARLIE-MARIE
CHARLIE-MAY
CHARLIE-RAE
CHARLIE-RAY
CHARLIE-ROSE
CHARLIE-THOMAS
CHARLIEANN
CHARLIEE
CHARLIEGH
CHARLINA
CHARLINE
CHARLISE
CHARLIZE
CHARLOTTA
CHARLOTTE
CHARLOTTE-ANN
CHARLOTTE-ANNE
CHARLOTTE-LOUISE
CHARLOTTE-MAE
CHARLOTTE-MARIE
CHARLOTTE-MAY
CHARLOTTE-RAE
CHARLOTTE-ROSE
CHARLTON
CHARLY
CHARLYN
CHARM
CHARMAIN
CHARMAINE
CHARMI
CHARMIAN
CHARNA
CHARNAE
CHARNE

CHARNEL
CHARNELLE
CHARNEY
CHARNIE
CHARVI
CHARVIK
CHARYS
CHAS
CHASE
CHASEY
CHASKA
CHAUDHARY
CHAUDHRY
CHAUDRY
CHAUNCEY
CHAUNTELLE
CHAVA
CHAVE
CHAVEZ
CHAVI
CHAVY
CHAWAN
CHAY
CHAYA
CHAYANNE
CHAYCE
CHAYDEN
CHAYE
CHAYIM
CHAYLA
CHAYSE
CHAYTON
CHAZ
CHE
CHEICK
CHEIKH
CHELBIE
CHELBY
CHELCIE
CHELSEA
CHELSEA-ANN
CHELSEA-ANNE
CHELSEA-JADE
CHELSEA-LEA
CHELSEA-LEE
CHELSEA-LEIGH
CHELSEA-LOUISE
CHELSEA-MAI

CHELSEA-MARIE
CHELSEA-MAY
CHELSEE
CHELSEY
CHELSEY-LEIGH
CHELSEY-MAY
CHELSI
CHELSIE
CHELSIE-LOUISE
CHELSY
CHEN
CHENAE
CHENAI
CHENAY
CHENAYA
CHENAYE
CHENE
CHENELLE
CHENG
CHENI
CHENICE
CHENILLE
CHENISE
CHENNAI
CHENOA
CHER
CHERAE
CHEREE
CHERELLE
CHERI
CHERICE
CHERIDAN
CHERIE
CHERIECE
CHERILYN
CHERISE
CHERISH
CHERISSE
CHERNICE
CHERNO
CHEROKEE
CHERRELLE
CHERRI
CHERRIE
CHERRY
CHERRY-LEIGH
CHERRY-ROSE
CHERYL

CHESKA	CHIEDOZIE	CHIRAG
CHESKEL	CHIEDZA	CHIRON
CHESKY	CHIEF	CHISIMDI
CHESNA	CHIEMEKA	CHISOM
CHESNEY	CHIEMENA	CHIYO
CHESTER	CHIGOZIE	CHIZARA
CHET	CHIGOZIRIM	CHIZARAM
CHETAN	CHIJIOKE	CHIZITARA
CHETNA	CHIKA	CHIZITELU
CHEUK	CHIKAIMA	CHIZITERE
CHEVELLE	CHIKAMSO	CHLOE
CHEVON	CHIKE	CHLOE-
CHEVONNE	CHIKEZIE	CHLOE-ANN
CHEVY	CHILLI	CHLOE-ANNE
CHEY	CHIMA	CHLOE-GRACE
CHEYA	CHIMAMANDA	CHLOE-JADE
CHEYANNA	CHIMAOBI	CHLOE-JANE
CHEYANNE	CHIMAOBIM	CHLOE-JAYNE
CHEYENNE	CHIMDINDU	CHLOE-JEAN
CHEYNE	CHIME	CHLOE-JO
CHEZNEY	CHIMEREMEZE	CHLOE-LEE
CHHAYA	CHIMNEDUM	CHLOE-LEIGH
CHI	CHINA	CHLOE-LOUISE
CHIA	CHINAZA	CHLOE-MAE
CHIAGOZIEM	CHINEDU	CHLOE-MAI
CHIAMAKA	CHINEDUM	CHLOE-MARIE
CHIAMANDA	CHINELO	CHLOE-MAY
CHIANA	CHINEMELUM	CHLOE-NICOLE
CHIANNA	CHINEMEREM	CHLOE-PAIGE
CHIANNE	CHINENYE	CHLOE-RAE
CHIARA	CHING	CHLOE-ROSE
CHIBUEZE	CHINMAYI	CHLOE-SOPHIA
CHIBUIKE	CHINO	CHLOEE
CHIBUIKEM	CHINOMSO	CHLOEY
CHIBUZO	CHINONSO	CHLOIE
CHICO	CHINONYE	CHOI
CHIDERA	CHINONYELUM	CHOLE
CHIDI	CHINONYEREM	CHONTELLE
CHIDIEBERE	CHINUA	CHOUDARY
CHIDIEBUBE	CHINUALUMOGU	CHOUDHARY
CHIDIMA	CHINWE	CHOUDHRY
CHIDIMMA	CHINWENDU	CHOUDHURY
CHIDINDU	CHINYERE	CHOWDHURY
CHIDINMA	CHIOMA	CHRA
CHIDO	CHIONE	CHRIS
CHIDOZIE	CHIPO	CHRIS-JUNIOR
CHIDUBEM	CHIQUITA	CHRISSIE
CHIDUMEBI	CHIRAAG	CHRISSY

CHRIST	CHUKWUKA	CIHAN
CHRISTA	CHUKWUMA	CILLIAN
CHRISTABEL	CHUKWUNONSO	CINAR
CHRISTABELLE	CHUMA	CINDY
CHRISTAKIS	CHUN	CINZIA
CHRISTAL	CHUNG	CION
CHRISTALLA	CHURCHILL	CIONA
CHRISTAN	CHYAN	CIRA
CHRISTEL	CHYANN	CIRAN
CHRISTELLE	CHYANNA	CIRO
CHRISTEN	CHYANNE	CIRON
CHRISTI	CHYENNE	CISSY
CHRISTIAAN	CHYNA	CIVAN
CHRISTIAN	CHYNA-ROSE	CIWAN
CHRISTIANA	CHYNNA	CIYA
CHRISTIANAH	CIA	CJ
CHRISTIANE	CIABHAN	CJAY
CHRISTIANNA	CIAN	CLAIR
CHRISTIANNE	CIANA	CLAIRA
CHRISTIANO	CIANAN	CLAIRE
CHRISTIE	CIANN	CLAIRE-LOUISE
CHRISTIEN	CIANNA	CLAITON
CHRISTINA	CIANNE	CLANCY
CHRISTINE	CIAR	CLARA
CHRISTO	CIARA	CLARA-ROSE
CHRISTOFER	CIARA-LEIGH	CLARABELLE
CHRISTOFF	CIARAH	CLARE
CHRISTOFOROS	CIARAN	CLARENCE
CHRISTON	CIAREN	CLARICE
CHRISTOPH	CIARNA	CLARIS
CHRISTOPHE	CIARON	CLARISA
CHRISTOPHER	CIARRA	CLARISE
CHRISTOPHER-JAMES	CICELY	CLARISSA
CHRISTOPHER-JAY	CICI	CLARISSE
CHRISTOPHER-JOHN	CICILY	CLARK
CHRISTOPHER-JUNIOR	CIDNEY	CLARKE
CHRISTOS	CIEANNA	CLARRISA
CHRISTVIE	CIEL	CLAUDE
CHRISTY	CIELO	CLAUDETTE
CHRYSTAL	CIENA	CLAUDIA
CHRYSTELLE	CIENNA	CLAUDIE
CHUKA	CIENNA-ROSE	CLAUDINE
CHUKWUBUIKEM	CIERA	CLAUDIO
CHUKWUDI	CIERAN	CLAUDIU
CHUKWUDUBEM	CIEREN	CLAUDIUS
CHUKWUDUMEBI	CIERON	CLAY
CHUKWUEBUKA	CIERRA	CLAYDON
CHUKWUEMEKA	CIGDEM	CLAYTON

CLEA
CLEM
CLEMENCE
CLEMENCIE
CLEMENCY
CLEMENT
CLEMENTINA
CLEMENTINE
CLEMMIE
CLEO
CLEO-ROSE
CLEON
CLEONA
CLEOPATRA
CLEVELAND
CLIFF
CLIFFORD
CLIFTON
CLINT
CLINTON
CLIO
CLIODHNA
CLIONA
CLIRIM
CLIVE
CLODAGH
CLODIE
CLOE
CLOEY
CLOIE
CLOTILDE
CLOUD
CLOVE
CLOVER
CLOVIS
CLYDE
COADY
COAN
COAST
COBAIN
COBAN
COBEN
COBEY
COBI
COBIE
COBURN
COBY
COBY-JAMES

COBY-JAY
COBY-LEE
COBY-RAY
COBYN
COCO
CODA
CODEE
CODEI
CODEN
CODEY
CODEY-LEE
CODI
CODIE
CODIE-JAMES
CODIE-LEIGH
CODY
CODY-JAMES
CODY-JAY
CODY-LEE
CODY-RAY
COEL
COEN
COFI
COHAN
COHAN-JAY
COHEN
COLBEY
COLBIE
COLBY
COLBY-LEE
COLE
COLE-JAMES
COLEBY
COLEEN
COLETON
COLETTE
COLEY
COLIN
COLLEEN
COLLETTE
COLLIN
COLLINS
COLM
COLT
COLTON
COLTRANE
COLUM
COLUMBUS

COLWYN
COMFORT
CONAGH
CONAH
CONAILL
CONAL
CONALL
CONAN
CONAR
CONAUGH
CONCETTA
CONDOLEEZZA
CONER
CONIE
CONLAN
CONLEY
CONN
CONNA
CONNAGH
CONNAH
CONNAIRE
CONNAL
CONNALL
CONNAN
CONNAR
CONNEL
CONNELL
CONNER
CONNER-LEE
CONNI
CONNIE
CONNIE-LEIGH
CONNIE-LOUISE
CONNIE-MAE
CONNIE-MAI
CONNIE-MARIE
CONNIE-MAY
CONNIE-RAE
CONNIE-ROSE
CONNOR
CONNOR-JAMES
CONNOR-JAY
CONNOR-JOE
CONNOR-LEE
CONNORLEE
CONNY
CONOR
CONOR-JAMES

CONRAD
CONRAN
CONROY
CONSTANCA
CONSTANCE
CONSTANDINA
CONSTANTIA
CONSTANTIN
CONSTANTINA
CONSTANTINE
CONSTANTINO
CONSTANTINOS
CONSTANZA
CONSUELA
CONWAY
COOPER
COOPER-JAMES
CORA
CORA-LEIGH
CORA-MAE
CORA-RAE
CORAH
CORAL
CORAL-ANNE
CORALE
CORALENA
CORALIE
CORALINE
CORAN
CORBAN
CORBEN
CORBIE
CORBIN
CORBON
CORBURN
CORBY
CORBYN
CORDAE
CORDE
CORDEL
CORDELIA
CORDELL
CORDEN
COREE
CORELLE
COREN
COREY
COREY-JAMES

COREY-JAY
COREY-LEE
COREY-LEIGH
COREY-TAYLOR
CORI
CORIE
CORIN
CORINA
CORINNA
CORINNE
CORLEY
CORMAC
CORMACK
CORNEL
CORNELIA
CORNELIUS
CORNELL
CORRA
CORRADO
CORRAN
CORREN
CORREY
CORRI
CORRIE
CORRIN
CORRINA
CORRINE
CORRINNE
CORRON
CORRY
CORRYN
CORTEZ
CORTNEY
CORTNIE
CORUM
CORVIN
CORWIN
CORY
CORY-LEE
CORYN
COSETTE
COSIMA
COSIMO
COSKUN
COSMIN
COSMINA
COSMO
COSMOS

COSTA
COSTANTINO
COSTANZA
COSTAS
COULTON
COUNTESS
COURAGE
COURTENAY
COURTENEY
COURTNAY
COURTNEE
COURTNEY
COURTNEY-
COURTNEY-JADE
COURTNEY-JANE
COURTNEY-JAYNE
COURTNEY-JO
COURTNEY-LEA
COURTNEY-LEE
COURTNEY-LEIGH
COURTNEY-LOUISE
COURTNEY-MAE
COURTNEY-MARIE
COURTNEY-MAY
COURTNEY-PAIGE
COURTNEY-ROSE
COURTNI
COURTNIE
COURTNY
COVE
COVEY
COWAN
COWEN
CRAIG
CRAIG-JUNIOR
CRAWFORD
CREE
CREED
CREEGAN
CRESSIDA
CREW
CREWE
CRIMEA
CRIMSON
CRINA
CRIS
CRISPIN
CRISTA

CRISTABEL
CRISTAL
CRISTELLE
CRISTIAN
CRISTIANA
CRISTIANO
CRISTINA
CRISTOBAL
CRISTOPHER
CRISTY
CROSBY
CROYDE
CRUE
CRUISE
CRUIZ
CRUIZE
CRUZ
CRUZE
CRYSTA
CRYSTABEL
CRYSTAL
CRYSTAL-ROSE
CRYSTEL
CRYSTELLE
CSABA
CSENGE
CSILLA
CSONGOR
CUAN
CUBA
CUBAN
CUINN
CULLAN
CULLEN
CULLUM
CULLY
CUMA
CURRAN
CURT
CURTIS
CURTIS-LEE
CURTISS
CURTLY
CUSHLA
CUTHBERT
CY
CYAN
CYANNA

CYANNE
CYD
CYDNEE
CYDNEY
CYDNI
CYDNIE
CYLE
CYNAN
CYNTHIA
CYPRIAN
CYPRIEN
CYPRUS
CYRA
CYRAN
CYRIL
CYRINE
CYRON
CYRUS
CYRYL

D

D
D'
D'ANDRE
D'ANGELO
D'ARCIE
D'ARCY
D'MARCO
D'MARI
D'SHAUN
DA
DA-XIA
DAAN
DAANIA
DAANISH
DAANIYA
DAANIYAL
DAANYA
DAANYAAL
DAANYAL
DABAN
DACEY
DACHI
DACIA
DACIAN
DACRE
DADE
DAEGAN
DAEJON
DAEMON
DAENA
DAENERYS
DAEVON
DAFFYD
DAFFYDD
DAFI
DAFINA
DAFNE
DAFYD
DAFYDD
DAGAN
DAGIM
DAGMARA
DAGMAWI
DAHA

DAHABO
DAHAT
DAHEN
DAHIR
DAHLIA
DAHNISH
DAI
DAIANA
DAICHI
DAIJA
DAIJON
DAIM
DAIMON
DAIN
DAINA
DAINE
DAINTON
DAIRE
DAISEE
DAISEY
DAISHA
DAISI
DAISIE
DAISIE-MAE
DAISIE-MAI
DAISIE-MAY
DAISIE-RAE
DAISY
DAISY-
DAISY-ANN
DAISY-ANNE
DAISY-BEAU
DAISY-BELLE
DAISY-BO
DAISY-BOO
DAISY-GRACE
DAISY-JADE
DAISY-JANE
DAISY-JAY
DAISY-JAYNE
DAISY-JO
DAISY-LEA
DAISY-LEE
DAISY-LEIGH
DAISY-LOU
DAISY-LOUISE
DAISY-MAE
DAISY-MAI

DAISY-MARIE
DAISY-MAY
DAISY-RAE
DAISY-ROSE
DAISY-SUE
DAISYMAY
DAITHI
DAITON
DAIVIK
DAIWIK
DAIYA
DAIYAAN
DAIYAN
DAIZIE
DAIZY
DAJAN
DAJANA
DAJUAN
DAKARAI
DAKODA
DAKOTA
DAKOTA-ROSE
DAKOTAH
DAKSH
DAKSHA
DALAL
DALANDA
DALE
DALEEP
DALEY
DALHA
DALI
DALIA
DALIAH
DALIAN
DALILA
DALILAH
DALISHA
DALIYA
DALIYAH
DALJINDER
DALJIT
DALLAN
DALLAS
DALRAJ
DALTON
DALVIN
DALVINDER

DALVIR
DALYA
DALZIEL
DAMAN
DAMANDEEP
DAMANI
DAMANPREET
DAMANVEER
DAMAR
DAMARAE
DAMARI
DAMARIO
DAMARION
DAMARIS
DAMARISA
DAMARLEY
DAMARNI
DAMEER
DAMEON
DAMIA
DAMIAN
DAMIANA
DAMIANO
DAMIEN
DAMIKA
DAMILARE
DAMILOLA
DAMINI
DAMION
DAMIR
DAMITA
DAMLA
DAMON
DAN
DANA
DANAE
DANAH
DANAI
DANAIL
DANAIT
DANANN
DANAR
DANAS
DANAYA
DANE
DANEEL
DANEEN
DANEIL

DANEKA
DANEL
DANELLA
DANELLE
DANER
DANESH
DANETTE
DANI
DANI-LEIGH
DANIA
DANIAAL
DANIAH
DANIAL
DANICA
DANIEL
DANIEL-JAMES
DANIEL-JOSEPH
DANIEL-JUNIOR
DANIEL-LEE
DANIELA
DANIELE
DANIELIS
DANIELIUS
DANIELLA
DANIELLE
DANIELS
DANII
DANIIL
DANIILS
DANIKA
DANIL
DANILA
DANILO
DANIQUE
DANIS
DANISH
DANISHA
DANITA
DANIYA
DANIYAAL
DANIYAH
DANIYAL
DANNA
DANNAN
DANNI
DANNI-LEIGH
DANNI-MARIE
DANNICA

DANNIE
DANNIEL
DANNIELLA
DANNIELLE
DANNII
DANNII-LEIGH
DANNIKA
DANNISH
DANNON
DANNY
DANNY-JAMES
DANNY-JAY
DANNY-JOE
DANNY-JUNIOR
DANNY-LEE
DANNYLEE
DANSON
DANTAE
DANTAY
DANTE
DANUJAN
DANUSH
DANUSHAN
DANUT
DANUTA
DANVEER
DANVIR
DANY
DANYA
DANYAAL
DANYAH
DANYAL
DANYAR
DANYEL
DANYELLE
DANYL
DANYLO
DAOOD
DAOUD
DAOUDA
DAPHNA
DAPHNE
DAPHNEY
DAQUAN
DARA
DARAGH
DARAH
DARASIMI

DARBY
DARCEE
DARCEY
DARCEY-LEE
DARCEY-LEIGH
DARCEY-MAE
DARCEY-MAI
DARCEY-MAY
DARCEY-RAE
DARCEY-ROSE
DARCI
DARCI-LEIGH
DARCI-MAE
DARCI-MAI
DARCI-MAY
DARCI-RAE
DARCI-ROSE
DARCIA
DARCIE
DARCIE-ANN
DARCIE-BEAU
DARCIE-GRACE
DARCIE-JANE
DARCIE-JO
DARCIE-LEA
DARCIE-LEIGH
DARCIE-LOUISE
DARCIE-MAE
DARCIE-MAI
DARCIE-MARIE
DARCIE-MAY
DARCIE-RAE
DARCIE-RAI
DARCIE-ROSE
DARCY
DARCY-ANN
DARCY-ELLA
DARCY-GRACE
DARCY-LEE
DARCY-LEIGH
DARCY-MAE
DARCY-MAI
DARCY-MARIE
DARCY-MAY
DARCY-RAE
DARCY-ROSE
DARDAN
DAREEN

DAREK
DARELL
DAREN
DARIA
DARIAN
DARIANA
DARIANNE
DARIEN
DARIJA
DARIM
DARIN
DARINA
DARINE
DARINKA
DARIO
DARION
DARIQ
DARIS
DARISHA
DARIUS
DARIUSH
DARIUSZ
DARIYA
DARIYAN
DARJA
DARLA
DARLA-RAE
DARLA-ROSE
DARLAH
DARLENE
DARLEY
DARLIA
DARLINGTON
DARNA
DARNEL
DARNELL
DARNELLE
DARO
DARON
DARRAGH
DARRAN
DARREL
DARRELL
DARREN
DARRIAN
DARRIEN
DARRIN
DARRION

DARRIUS
DARRON
DARRYL
DARRYLL
DARRYN
DARSH
DARSHAN
DARSHANA
DARSHI
DARSHIK
DARSHIL
DARSHINI
DARVIN
DARWIN
DARWYN
DARYA
DARYAN
DARYL
DARYLE
DARYLL
DARYN
DARYUS
DAS
DASH
DASHA
DASHAWN
DASHIEL
DASHIELL
DASIA
DASSY
DASTAN
DAUD
DAUDA
DAULTON
DAVANTE
DAVE
DAVEENA
DAVEN
DAVENA
DAVEY
DAVI
DAVIA
DAVIAN
DAVID
DAVID-JAMES
DAVID-JUNIOR
DAVID-LEE
DAVIDA

DAVIDAS	DAYYAN	DEE
DAVIDE	DE	DEE-JAY
DAVIDS	DE'	DEEA
DAVIDSON	DE'ANDRE	DEEANA
DAVIE	DE'ANGELO	DEEANNA
DAVIES	DE'SHAUN	DEEBA
DAVIN	DEA	DEEDEE
DAVINA	DEACAN	DEEGAN
DAVINDER	DEACON	DEEHAN
DAVINE	DEACON-JAMES	DEEJAY
DAVINIA	DEAGAN	DEEKSHA
DAVION	DEAGLAN	DEELAN
DAVIS	DEAGO	DEEM
DAVIT	DEAH	DEEMA
DAVITA	DEAKAN	DEEN
DAVON	DEAKEN	DEENA
DAVONTAE	DEAKIN	DEENAH
DAVONTE	DEAKON	DEEP
DAVUT	DEAN	DEEPA
DAVY	DEAN-JUNIOR	DEEPAK
DAWDA	DEANA	DEEPALI
DAWID	DEANDRA	DEEPESH
DAWIT	DEANDRE	DEEPIKA
DAWN	DEANE	DEEPTI
DAWOOD	DEANGELO	DEEQA
DAWOUD	DEANNA	DEESHA
DAWSON	DEANNA-MARIE	DEESHAN
DAWUD	DEANNE	DEETYA
DAX	DEANO	DEEVA
DAXTON	DEARBHLA	DEEWA
DAYA	DEBA	DEEYA
DAYAAN	DEBBIE	DEEYAN
DAYAL	DEBBY	DEFNE
DAYAN	DEBORA	DEIA
DAYANA	DEBORAH	DEIAN
DAYLA	DEBRA	DEIGHTON
DAYLAN	DEBRAH	DEIMANTAS
DAYLE	DECCA	DEIMANTE
DAYLEY	DECHLAN	DEINA
DAYNA	DECKLAN	DEINAS
DAYNE	DECKLAND	DEINIOL
DAYNTON	DECLAN	DEIO
DAYSHA	DECLAN-JAMES	DEION
DAYSHAUN	DECLAND	DEIRDRE
DAYSIE	DECLEN	DEITRICK
DAYTON	DECLYN	DEIVID
DAYTONA	DECON	DEIVIDAS
DAYYAAN	DEDAN	DEIVIDS

DEIVYDAS
DEJA
DEJAH
DEJAN
DEJANA
DEJANAE
DEJAUN
DEJAY
DEJEAN
DEJON
DEJOURN
DEJUAN
DEKA
DEKLAN
DEKLAND
DEKOTA
DEL
DELA
DELAL
DELAN
DELANA
DELANEY
DELANIE
DELANO
DELARA
DELCIA
DELCIE
DELENN
DELFINA
DELIA
DELICIA
DELIGHT
DELILA
DELILAH
DELILAH-MAE
DELILAH-MAY
DELILAH-RAE
DELILAH-ROSE
DELINA
DELISHA
DELLA
DELLAN
DELNA
DELON
DELORES
DELPHI
DELPHIE
DELPHINA

DELPHINE
DELROY
DELSA
DELSIE
DELTA
DELTON
DELUN
DELVIN
DELWYN
DELYLAH
DELYTH
DEMA
DEMANI
DEMAR
DEMARCO
DEMARI
DEMARIO
DEMARNI
DEMBA
DEMEE
DEMELZA
DEMET
DEMETRA
DEMETRI
DEMETRIA
DEMETRIOS
DEMETRIS
DEMETRIUS
DEMI
DEMI-
DEMI-ANN
DEMI-ANNE
DEMI-ELISE
DEMI-GRACE
DEMI-JADE
DEMI-JAY
DEMI-JO
DEMI-LEA
DEMI-LEE
DEMI-LEI
DEMI-LEIGH
DEMI-LOU
DEMI-LOUISE
DEMI-MAE
DEMI-MAI
DEMI-MARIE
DEMI-MAY
DEMI-NICOLE

DEMI-RAE
DEMI-ROSE
DEMIAN
DEMID
DEMIE
DEMIE-LEIGH
DEMII
DEMILADE
DEMILEA
DEMILEE
DEMILEIGH
DEMILOUISE
DEMIR
DEMIRA
DEMISHA
DEMITRA
DEMITRI
DEMITRIA
DEMITRIUS
DEMMI
DEMMIE
DEMPSEY
DEMPSIE
DEN
DENA
DENAE
DENAN
DENAS
DENAYA
DENBY
DENE
DENELLE
DENES
DENHAM
DENHOLM
DENI
DENIA
DENICA
DENICE
DENIEL
DENIKA
DENIL
DENILSON
DENIM
DENIQUE
DENIRO
DENIS
DENISA

DENISE
DENISHA
DENISLAV
DENISS
DENIZ
DENLEY
DENNA
DENNAN
DENNI
DENNIE
DENNIS
DENNISON
DENNON
DENNY
DENON
DENTON
DENUM
DENVA
DENVER
DENYS
DENZEL
DENZELL
DENZIEL
DENZIL
DENZYL
DEO
DEON
DEONA
DEONDRE
DEONNE
DEONTAE
DEONTAY
DEONTE
DEQA
DEQUAN
DERAN
DERAY
DERECK
DEREECE
DEREK
DEREN
DERI
DERIAN
DERICE
DERICK
DERIN
DERMOT
DERON

DERRAN
DERRELL
DERREN
DERRI
DERRICK
DERRIE
DERRIN
DERRON
DERRY
DERRYN
DERVIS
DERVLA
DERWYN
DERYA
DERYN
DES'REE
DESARA
DESCHANEL
DESEAN
DESERAE
DESHAAN
DESHAN
DESHANE
DESHARN
DESHAUN
DESHAWN
DESHNA
DESHON
DESIRE
DESIREE
DESMOND
DESPINA
DESREE
DESTAN
DESTANY
DESTIN
DESTINA
DESTINE
DESTINEE
DESTINEY
DESTINI
DESTINIE
DESTINY
DESTINY-LOUISE
DESTINY-MAI
DESTINY-MARIE
DESTINY-MAY
DESTINY-RAE

DESTINY-ROSE
DETROY
DEUEL
DEV
DEVA
DEVAANSH
DEVAK
DEVAM
DEVAN
DEVANG
DEVANI
DEVANSH
DEVANSHI
DEVANTE
DEVARN
DEVARSH
DEVAUNTE
DEVEN
DEVESH
DEVI
DEVIKA
DEVIN
DEVINA
DEVINDER
DEVINE
DEVISHA
DEVLIN
DEVLYN
DEVNA
DEVOIRY
DEVON
DEVONDRE
DEVONNE
DEVONTA
DEVONTAE
DEVONTAI
DEVONTAY
DEVONTE
DEVORA
DEVORAH
DEVRAJ
DEVRAN
DEVRIM
DEVUN
DEVYAN
DEVYN
DEWAN
DEWAYNE

DEWI	DHIAAN	DIANTE
DEX	DHIAN	DIAR
DEXI	DHILAN	DIARMAID
DEXIE	DHILLAN	DIARMUID
DEXTER	DHILLON	DIAVIAN
DEXTER-JAMES	DHILON	DIAZ
DEXY	DHIR	DIBA
DEYA	DHIRAJ	DIBORA
DEYAAN	DHIREN	DICKSON
DEYAN	DHIYA	DICLE
DEYANA	DHIYAAN	DIDAR
DHAANI	DHIYAN	DIDEM
DHAIRYA	DHOHA	DIDI
DHALIA	DHRISH	DIDIER
DHANANJAY	DHRITI	DIEGO
DHANESH	DHRIYA	DIELLZA
DHANI	DHRU	DIESEL
DHANIAL	DHRUTI	DIETER
DHANISH	DHRUV	DIEUDONNE
DHANISHA	DHRUVA	DIEZEL
DHANISHTA	DHRUVAN	DIGBY
DHANIYAL	DHRUVI	DIGGORY
DHANRAJ	DHRUVIKA	DIGORY
DHANUSH	DHRUVIN	DIHAIN
DHANVEER	DHRUVISHA	DIHEIN
DHANVI	DHUHA	DIJA
DHANVIN	DHVANI	DIJLE
DHANYA	DHWANI	DIJON
DHANYAAL	DHYAAN	DIKSHA
DHANYAL	DHYAN	DILA
DHARA	DHYANA	DILAKSHAN
DHARAM	DHYANI	DILAKSHIKA
DHARAMVEER	DHYEY	DILAN
DHARM	DHYLAN	DILANA
DHARMA	DIA	DILANAS
DHARMESH	DIAGO	DILANI
DHARMIK	DIAKO	DILANS
DHARSHAN	DIALA	DILARA
DHARSHINI	DIALLO	DILAWAR
DHARUN	DIAMANT	DILAY
DHAVAL	DIAMOND	DILEEP
DHAVAN	DIAN	DILEK
DHAVINA	DIANA	DILEM
DHAYA	DIANDRA	DILEN
DHEEN	DIANDRE	DILESH
DHEER	DIANE	DILETA
DHEERAN	DIANNA	DILHAN
DHEVAN	DIANNE	DILIP

DILJOT	DIONYSUS	DIYARI
DILLAN	DIOR	DIYON
DILLEN	DIORA	DJ
DILLION	DIPALI	DJAMEL
DILLON	DIPESH	DJAMILA
DILLY	DIPIKA	DJANGO
DILON	DIPSON	DJELLONA
DILPREET	DIQUAN	DJELLZA
DILRAAJ	DIREN	DJIBRIL
DILRAJ	DIRK	DJIMON
DILREET	DISA	DJORDJE
DILSHAAN	DISHA	DJUNA
DILSHAN	DISHAAN	DMITRI
DILVEER	DISHAN	DMITRIJ
DILWAR	DISHITA	DMITRIJS
DILYS	DISNEY	DMITRIY
DIMA	DITA	DMITRY
DIMITAR	DITHUSAN	DMYTRO
DIMITRA	DITI	DOAA
DIMITRI	DIVA	DODI
DIMITRIE	DIVAM	DOGA
DIMITRIJE	DIVESH	DOGAN
DIMITRIOS	DIVIJ	DOGUKAN
DIMITRIS	DIVIN	DOGUS
DIMPLE	DIVINA	DOHA
DIN	DIVINE	DOHYUN
DINA	DIVISHA	DOLAPO
DINAH	DIVIT	DOLCE
DINARA	DIVJOT	DOLCEE
DINARI	DIVLEEN	DOLCEY
DINEL	DIVYA	DOLCI
DINESH	DIVYAM	DOLCIE
DINI	DIVYAN	DOLCIE-LOU
DINIS	DIVYANKA	DOLCIE-MAE
DINITHI	DIVYANSH	DOLCIE-MAI
DINO	DIVYANSHI	DOLCIE-MAY
DINUK	DIVYESH	DOLCIE-RAE
DINUKI	DIWAN	DOLLI
DIOGO	DIXIE	DOLLIE
DION	DIXIE-MAE	DOLLIE-MAE
DIONA	DIXON	DOLLIE-MAI
DIONDRE	DIYA	DOLLIE-RAE
DIONE	DIYAAN	DOLLIE-ROSE
DIONIS	DIYAKO	DOLLY
DIONISIO	DIYAN	DOLLY-ANN
DIONNE	DIYANA	DOLLY-ANNA
DIONTAE	DIYANAH	DOLLY-MAE
DIONTE	DIYAR	DOLLY-MAI

DOLLY-MARIE	DONE	DOTTY
DOLLY-MAY	DONELL	DOTTY-ROSE
DOLLY-RAE	DONELLA	DOUAA
DOLLY-ROSE	DONELLE	DOUG
DOLLYANNA	DONG	DOUGAL
DOLORES	DONI	DOUGIE
DOLSIE	DONIA	DOUGLAS
DOLTON	DONIEL	DOULTON
DOMANIC	DONIKA	DOUNIA
DOMANTAS	DONJETA	DOV
DOMAS	DONNA	DOVAS
DOMENIC	DONNA-MARIE	DOVI
DOMENICA	DONNACHA	DOVID
DOMENICO	DONNCHA	DOVIDAS
DOMENIK	DONNEL	DOVYDAS
DOMENIKS	DONNELL	DOYINSOLA
DOMINI	DONNIE	DOYLE
DOMINIC	DONNY	DRACO
DOMINIC-JOHN	DONOVAN	DRAE
DOMINICA	DONTA	DRAGAN
DOMINICK	DONTAE	DRAGOS
DOMINIK	DONTAI	DRAKE
DOMINIKA	DONTAY	DRASHTI
DOMINIKAS	DONTAYE	DRAVEN
DOMINIKS	DONTE	DRAVID
DOMINION	DONYA	DRAY
DOMINIQUE	DORA	DRAYDEN
DOMINO	DORAN	DRAZIC
DOMINYKA	DORCAS	DRE
DOMINYKAS	DOREEN	DREAM
DOMONIC	DORIAN	DREN
DOMONIQUE	DORINA	DRENUSHA
DON	DORINDA	DREW
DONA	DORIS	DREY
DONAE	DORKA	DREYA
DONAEO	DORNA	DRIES
DONAL	DORON	DRILON
DONALD	DOROTA	DRIN
DONART	DOROTHEA	DRINA
DONAT	DOROTHY	DRINI
DONATA	DOROTTYA	DRISHTI
DONATAS	DORRELL	DRISS
DONATELLA	DORRIAN	DRITI
DONATELLO	DORSA	DROOD
DONATO	DORUK	DRU
DONAVAN	DOTTI	DRUE
DONAVON	DOTTIE	DRUMMOND
DONDU	DOTTIE-MAE	DRUSILLA

DRUV
DRYDEN
DRYSTAN
DUA
DUAA
DUAINE
DUANA
DUANE
DUANE-LEE
DUARTE
DUBEM
DUC
DUCHESS
DUDLEY
DUHA
DUKE
DULCE
DULCIE
DULCIMA
DUMITRU
DUNCAN
DUNIA
DUNYA
DURAN
DURELL
DURGA
DURIEL
DURMUS
DURRE
DURRELL
DURSUN
DURU
DUSAN
DUSTIN
DUSTY
DUTCH
DUVAL
DUVALL
DUWA
DUY
DUYGU
DVITI
DWAIN
DWAINE
DWAYNE
DWIGHT
DWIJ
DWYNWEN

DYA
DYAKO
DYANI
DYFAN
DYFED
DYLAN
DYLAN-JAMES
DYLAN-JOHN
DYLAN-LEE
DYLAN-RHYS
DYLAN-THOMAS
DYLANN
DYLEN
DYLIS
DYLLAN
DYLLON
DYLON
DYNASTY
DYRELL
DYSON
DZESIKA
DZIFA
DZIUGAS

E

EABHA
EADEE
EADEN
EADIE
EADIE-ROSE
EADY
EAGAN
EALAF
EAMON
EAMONN
EANNA
EARL
EARNEST
EARTHA
EASA
EASAH
EASHA
EASHAN
EASHAR
EASHEN
EASHER
EASON
EASTER
EASTON
EATHAN
EATHEN
EAVAN
EAVIE
EBADUR
EBAN
EBANIE
EBANY
EBBA
EBBEN
EBBIE
EBBONIE
EBEN
EBENEZER
EBON
EBONEE
EBONEY
EBONI
EBONIE
EBONIE-MAI

EBONIE-ROSE
EBONNIE
EBONY
EBONY-
EBONY-GRACE
EBONY-JADE
EBONY-LEIGH
EBONY-LOUISE
EBONY-MAE
EBONY-MAI
EBONY-MAY
EBONY-RAE
EBONY-ROSE
EBRAHEEM
EBRAHIM
EBRAR
EBRIMA
EBRU
EBUBECHI
EBUBECHUKWU
EBUBEKIR
EBUNOLUWA
EBUWA
EBYAN
ECATERINA
ECE
ECEM
ECENAZ
ECHO
ECRIN
ECTOR
ED
EDA
EDAN
EDAS
EDDI
EDDIE
EDDIE-JAMES
EDDISON
EDDY
EDE
EDEE
EDEL
EDELE
EDEM
EDEN
EDEN-GRACE
EDEN-JAMES

EDEN-LEIGH
EDEN-LILY
EDEN-MAE
EDEN-RAE
EDEN-ROSE
EDEY
EDGAR
EDGARAS
EDGARS
EDI
EDIE
EDIE-BELLE
EDIE-MAE
EDIE-MAY
EDIE-ROSE
EDIJS
EDIL
EDIN
EDINA
EDION
EDIS
EDISON
EDITA
EDITH
EDITH-MAY
EDITH-ROSE
EDIZ
EDLYN
EDMOND
EDMUND
EDNA
EDOARDO
EDOM
EDON
EDONA
EDONIS
EDOSA
EDOUARD
EDRIC
EDRIS
EDSON
EDUARD
EDUARDA
EDUARDO
EDUARDS
EDUART
EDVARD
EDVARDAS

EDVARDS
EDVIN
EDVINAS
EDWARD
EDWARD-JAMES
EDWIN
EDWINA
EDWYN
EDY
EDYN
EDYTA
EDYTH
EDYTHE
EEDIE
EEMAAN
EEMAN
EEQAN
EEREN
EESA
EESAA
EESAH
EESHA
EESHAL
EESHAN
EESSA
EETHAN
EEVA
EEVEE
EEVIE
EFA
EFAN
EFAZ
EFE
EFEMENA
EFETOBORE
EFEZINO
EFFI
EFFIA
EFFIE
EFFIE-MAE
EFFIE-ROSE
EFFY
EFIA
EFOSA
EFRAIM
EFRAN
EFRATA
EFREM

EFREN
EFSA
EFTELYA
EFUA
EGAN
EGE
EGHOSA
EGLE
EGOR
EGYPT
EGZON
EGZONA
EHAAN
EHAB
EHAN
EHLANA
EHREN
EHSAAN
EHSAN
EHSANUL
EHSEN
EHTESHAM
EHTISHAM
EIBHLEANN
EIBHLIN
EIBHLINN
EID
EIDAN
EIDANAS
EIDEN
EIDENAS
EIDY
EIFA
EIFION
EIJAZ
EIJI
EIKI
EILA
EILA-ROSE
EILAH
EILEEN
EILIDH
EILIR
EILIS
EILISH
EILIYA
EILIYAH
EILY

EIMAAN
EIMAN
EIMANTAS
EIMEAR
EIMER
EIMILE
EINAR
EINION
EINORAS
EIRA
EIRE
EIREANN
EIREN
EIRENE
EIRI
EIRIAN
EIRIANWEN
EIRIK
EIRIN
EIRINI
EIRINN
EIRLYS
EIRWEN
EIRY
EIRYN
EIRYS
EISA
EISAA
EISAH
EISHA
EISSA
EISUKE
EITA
EITAN
EITHAN
EITHNE
EITO
EIVA
EIVIN
EIVISSA
EJAZ
EJIRO
EJONA
EKAM
EKAMDEEP
EKAMJEET
EKAMJIT
EKAMJOT

EKAMPREET	ELAYA	ELENI
EKAMVEER	ELAYAH	ELENID
EKANSH	ELAYNA	ELENIE
EKATERINA	ELBA	ELENNA
EKATERINI	ELBIE	ELENOR
EKENE	ELCHONON	ELENORA
EKHUM	ELCIE	ELENORE
EKIN	ELDA	ELENYA
EKKAM	ELDAD	ELEONOR
EKLAVYA	ELDANA	ELEONORA
EKNOOR	ELDAR	ELEONORE
EKOW	ELDEN	ELEORA
EKRAM	ELDI	ELERI
EKREM	ELDIN	ELESA
EKROOP	ELDON	ELESE
EKTA	ELDRIDGE	ELESHA
EKTOR	ELEA	ELETTRA
EKTORAS	ELEAH	ELEXA
EKUNDAYO	ELEANA	ELEXIA
EL	ELEANER	ELEXIE
ELA	ELEANNA	ELEXIS
ELA-MAI	ELEANOR	ELEXUS
ELAAF	ELEANOR-MAE	ELEYANA
ELADA	ELEANOR-MAY	ELEYNA
ELAF	ELEANOR-ROSE	ELFIDA
ELAH	ELEANORA	ELFIE
ELAHA	ELEANORE	ELFIN
ELAI	ELEASHA	ELFINE
ELAIA	ELEAZAR	ELFREDA
ELAIN	ELECIA	ELGAN
ELAINA	ELECTRA	ELGIN
ELAINE	ELEEN	ELHAAM
ELAN	ELEENA	ELHADJ
ELANA	ELEESHA	ELHAM
ELANAH	ELEEZA	ELI
ELANAS	ELEFTHERIA	ELI-JAMES
ELANAZ	ELEIGH	ELIA
ELANI	ELEINA	ELIAB
ELANNA	ELEISHA	ELIAH
ELANO	ELEIYAH	ELIAKIM
ELANOR	ELEKTRA	ELIAM
ELANORE	ELELTA	ELIAN
ELANUR	ELEN	ELIANA
ELANYA	ELENA	ELIANAH
ELARA	ELENA-MAE	ELIANE
ELARNA	ELENA-MAY	ELIANNA
ELAURA	ELENA-ROSE	ELIANNE
ELAY	ELENE	ELIAS

ELIASZ
ELIAV
ELIAZER
ELICA
ELICE
ELICIA
ELIDA
ELIE
ELIEL
ELIESE
ELIESHA
ELIEZER
ELIF
ELIFNAZ
ELIFSU
ELIGH
ELIH
ELIJA
ELIJAH
ELIJAH-JAMES
ELIJAH-MOSES
ELIJAS
ELIJUS
ELIKA
ELIKEM
ELIM
ELIMELECH
ELIN
ELINA
ELINAM
ELINE
ELINOR
ELINORE
ELIO
ELIOENAI
ELION
ELIONA
ELIORA
ELIOS
ELIOT
ELIOTT
ELIRA
ELIS
ELISA
ELISABET
ELISABETA
ELISABETH
ELISABETTA

ELISAVETA
ELISE
ELISEI
ELISEO
ELISH
ELISHA
ELISHA-MAI
ELISHA-MARIE
ELISHA-MAY
ELISHEBA
ELISHEVA
ELISHIA
ELISHKA
ELISIA
ELISKA
ELISSA
ELISSA-MAE
ELISSE
ELISSIA
ELISSIA-ROSE
ELITA
ELITHEA
ELITSA
ELIUD
ELIVIA
ELIYA
ELIYAH
ELIYAHU
ELIYANA
ELIYANAH
ELIYAS
ELIYOHU
ELIZ
ELIZA
ELIZA-ANN
ELIZA-GRACE
ELIZA-JANE
ELIZA-JEAN
ELIZA-LILLY
ELIZA-LILY
ELIZA-LOUISE
ELIZA-MAE
ELIZA-MAI
ELIZA-MAY
ELIZA-RAE
ELIZA-ROSE
ELIZABELLA
ELIZABET

ELIZABETA
ELIZABETE
ELIZABETH
ELIZABETH-ANN
ELIZABETH-GRACE
ELIZABETH-MAY
ELIZABETH-ROSE
ELIZAH
ELIZAVETA
ELIZE
ELJAY
ELJON
ELKA
ELKAN
ELKANAH
ELKE
ELKIE
ELLA
ELLA-
ELLA-ANN
ELLA-ANNE
ELLA-BROOKE
ELLA-FAITH
ELLA-GRACE
ELLA-JADE
ELLA-JAI
ELLA-JANE
ELLA-JAY
ELLA-JAYNE
ELLA-JEAN
ELLA-JO
ELLA-JOY
ELLA-KATE
ELLA-LEIGH
ELLA-LOUISE
ELLA-MAE
ELLA-MAI
ELLA-MARIA
ELLA-MARIE
ELLA-MAY
ELLA-NICOLE
ELLA-RAE
ELLA-RAI
ELLA-ROSE
ELLA-RUBY
ELLA-SOPHIA
ELLAH
ELLAINA

ELLALOUISE
ELLAMAE
ELLAMAY
ELLAN
ELLANA
ELLAND
ELLANOR
ELLANORE
ELLAOUISE
ELLARA
ELLARIA
ELLAROSE
ELLE
ELLE-
ELLE-ANN
ELLE-JANE
ELLE-JAY
ELLE-JO
ELLE-LEIGH
ELLE-LOUISE
ELLE-MAE
ELLE-MAI
ELLE-MARIE
ELLE-MAY
ELLE-ROSE
ELLEA
ELLEAH
ELLEANA
ELLEANNA
ELLEANOR
ELLECE
ELLECIA
ELLEE
ELLEECE
ELLEIGH
ELLEISE
ELLEISHA
ELLEMAE
ELLEMAY
ELLEN
ELLEN-ROSE
ELLENA
ELLENER
ELLENI
ELLENIE
ELLENOR
ELLERIE
ELLERY

ELLESE
ELLESHA
ELLESHIA
ELLESIA
ELLESSE
ELLESSIA
ELLEXIS
ELLEY
ELLI
ELLI-MAE
ELLI-MAI
ELLIA
ELLIAH
ELLIANA
ELLIANNA
ELLIANNE
ELLIAS
ELLICE
ELLICIA
ELLIE
ELLIE-
ELLIE-ANN
ELLIE-ANNA
ELLIE-ANNE
ELLIE-BROOKE
ELLIE-GRACE
ELLIE-J
ELLIE-JADE
ELLIE-JAE
ELLIE-JAI
ELLIE-JANE
ELLIE-JAY
ELLIE-JAYNE
ELLIE-JEAN
ELLIE-JO
ELLIE-KAY
ELLIE-LEIGH
ELLIE-LOU
ELLIE-LOUISE
ELLIE-MAE
ELLIE-MAI
ELLIE-MAII
ELLIE-MARIE
ELLIE-MAY
ELLIE-MAYE
ELLIE-NICOLE
ELLIE-PAIGE
ELLIE-RAE

ELLIE-ROSE
ELLIE-SUE
ELLIEANN
ELLIEANNE
ELLIEMAE
ELLIEMAI
ELLIEMAY
ELLIEROSE
ELLIESE
ELLIESHA
ELLIETTE
ELLIJAH
ELLIN
ELLINA
ELLINOR
ELLIOT
ELLIOT-JAMES
ELLIOTT
ELLIOTT-JAMES
ELLIOTTE
ELLIS
ELLIS-JAMES
ELLIS-JAY
ELLISA
ELLISE
ELLISHA
ELLISHIA
ELLISIA
ELLISON
ELLISS
ELLISSA
ELLISSE
ELLISSIA
ELLIVIA
ELLIW
ELLIYA
ELLIYAH
ELLIZA
ELLOISE
ELLORA
ELLOUISA
ELLOUISE
ELLSA
ELLSEY
ELLSIE
ELLY
ELLY-MAE
ELLY-MAY

ELLYANA	ELSA	ELWEN
ELLYCE	ELSA-GRACE	ELWIN
ELLYCIA	ELSA-MAE	ELWOOD
ELLYN	ELSA-MAI	ELWYN
ELLYS	ELSA-MAY	ELY
ELLYSE	ELSA-ROSE	ELYA
ELLYSHA	ELSABETH	ELYAN
ELLYSIA	ELSBETH	ELYANA
ELLYSSA	ELSE	ELYAS
ELLYSSE	ELSEA	ELYCE
ELMA	ELSEE	ELYCIA
ELMAS	ELSEY	ELYES
ELMEDINA	ELSHADDAI	ELYN
ELMER	ELSI	ELYNOR
ELMI	ELSIE	ELYON
ELMIRA	ELSIE-ANN	ELYOTT
ELMO	ELSIE-ANNE	ELYS
ELMORE	ELSIE-BEAU	ELYSA
ELNA	ELSIE-BELLE	ELYSE
ELNATHAN	ELSIE-GRACE	ELYSHA
ELNAZ	ELSIE-JANE	ELYSHIA
ELOAH	ELSIE-JEAN	ELYSIA
ELODIE	ELSIE-LEIGH	ELYSIE
ELODIE-MAE	ELSIE-LOU	ELYSSA
ELODIE-ROSE	ELSIE-LOUISE	ELYSSE
ELODY	ELSIE-MAE	ELYSSIA
ELOGHOSA	ELSIE-MAI	ELYSTAN
ELOHIM	ELSIE-MARIE	ELYZA
ELOHOR	ELSIE-MAY	ELZA
ELOI	ELSIE-RAE	ELZBIETA
ELOISA	ELSIE-ROSE	ELZE
ELOISE	ELSIE-VIOLET	EMA
ELOISE-MAE	ELSIEMAE	EMAAD
ELON	ELSON	EMAAN
ELONA	ELSPETH	EMAANI
ELORA	ELSY	EMAD
ELORA-ROSE	ELTON	EMALEE
ELORM	ELULA	EMALEIGH
ELOUAN	ELUNED	EMALIE
ELOUISA	ELVA	EMAN
ELOUISE	ELVI	EMANI
ELOWEN	ELVIA	EMANUEL
ELOWYN	ELVIE	EMANUELA
ELOY	ELVIN	EMANUELE
ELOZOR	ELVINA	EMANUELLA
ELPHIE	ELVIRA	EMANUELLE
ELPIDA	ELVIS	EMARI
ELROY	ELVY	EMAYA

EMBER
EMBER-ROSE
EMBERLY
EMDADUL
EMDADUR
EME
EMEE
EMEFA
EMEILIA
EMEKA
EMEL
EMELDA
EMELI
EMELIA
EMELIA-GRACE
EMELIA-LILY
EMELIA-MAE
EMELIA-ROSE
EMELIAH
EMELIE
EMELINE
EMELLIA
EMELY
EMELYE
EMELYN
EMER
EMERALD
EMERIC
EMERIE
EMERITA
EMERSON
EMERY
EMESE
EMETAS
EMI
EMI-LEIGH
EMIE
EMIE-ROSE
EMIEL
EMIELIA
EMIKA
EMIKO
EMIL
EMILA
EMILE
EMILEA
EMILEE
EMILEE-ROSE

EMILEIGH
EMILEO
EMILEY
EMILI
EMILIA
EMILIA-GRACE
EMILIA-MAE
EMILIA-RAE
EMILIA-ROSE
EMILIAN
EMILIANA
EMILIANO
EMILIE
EMILIE-GRACE
EMILIE-JANE
EMILIE-MAE
EMILIE-MAY
EMILIE-ROSE
EMILIJA
EMILIJUS
EMILIO
EMILIOS
EMILIS
EMILIYA
EMILJA
EMILLIA
EMILLIE
EMILLY
EMILS
EMILY
EMILY-
EMILY-ANN
EMILY-ANNE
EMILY-ELIZABETH
EMILY-GRACE
EMILY-JADE
EMILY-JANE
EMILY-JAYNE
EMILY-JO
EMILY-KATE
EMILY-LOUISE
EMILY-MAE
EMILY-MAI
EMILY-MARIE
EMILY-MAY
EMILY-PAIGE
EMILY-RAE
EMILY-ROSE

EMILYA
EMILYJANE
EMILYROSE
EMIMA
EMIN
EMINA
EMINE
EMIOLA
EMIR
EMIRA
EMIRCAN
EMIRHAN
EMIS
EMLYN
EMMA
EMMA-
EMMA-GRACE
EMMA-JADE
EMMA-JANE
EMMA-JAYNE
EMMA-JO
EMMA-LEA
EMMA-LEE
EMMA-LEIGH
EMMA-LOUISE
EMMA-MARIE
EMMA-MAY
EMMA-ROSE
EMMALEE
EMMALEIGH
EMMALENE
EMMALINE
EMMALISE
EMMALOUISE
EMMALYN
EMMAN
EMMANOUIL
EMMANUAL
EMMANUEL
EMMANUELA
EMMANUELLA
EMMANUELLE
EMMAUNEL
EMME
EMMELIA
EMMELINE
EMMERSON
EMMET

EMMETT
EMMEY
EMMI
EMMI-LEIGH
EMMI-LOU
EMMI-LOUISE
EMMIE
EMMIE-GRACE
EMMIE-LEIGH
EMMIE-LOU
EMMIE-LOUISE
EMMIE-MAE
EMMIE-MAY
EMMIE-RAE
EMMIE-ROSE
EMMILY
EMMY
EMMY-LOU
EMMY-RAE
EMMYLOU
EMNA
EMNET
EMOGENE
EMON
EMORY
EMPRESS
EMRAH
EMRAN
EMRE
EMRYS
EMY
EMY-LEIGH
EMYLIA
EMYR
EN
ENA
ENAAYA
ENAIYA
ENAM
ENAMUL
ENARA
ENAS
ENAYA
ENAYAH
ENDA
ENDEAVOUR
ENDI
ENDIJA

ENDIJS
ENDRI
ENDRIT
ENEA
ENEIDA
ENES
ENESA
ENFYS
ENGIN
ENGJELL
ENID
ENIJA
ENIKO
ENIOLA
ENIOLUWA
ENIS
ENISA
ENISE
ENITAN
ENKI
ENLLI
ENNA
ENNIO
ENNIS
ENO
ENOCH
ENOCK
ENOH
ENOLA
ENORA
ENOSH
ENRI
ENRIC
ENRICO
ENRIK
ENRIKA
ENRIKAS
ENRIQUE
ENSAR
ENVER
ENXI
ENYA
ENYA-GRACE
ENYA-ROSE
ENZA
ENZI
ENZO
ENZZO

EOGHAN
EOIN
EOS
EOWYN
EPHIE
EPHRA
EPHRAIM
EPHRAM
EPHRATA
EPHREM
EPHRON
EPIPHANY
EPONINE
EPPIE
ERA
ERALD
ERALDA
ERALDO
ERAM
ERAN
ERAY
ERBLIN
ERCAN
ERDAL
ERDEM
ERDI
EREN
ERENCAN
ERESHVA
ERFAN
ERGI
ERGUN
ERGYS
ERHAN
ERI
ERIANA
ERIC
ERICA
ERICA-ROSE
ERICK
ERICKA
ERIDA
ERIK
ERIKA
ERIKAS
ERIKO
ERIKS
ERIM

ERIN
ERIN-
ERIN-GRACE
ERIN-LEIGH
ERIN-LILY
ERIN-LOUISE
ERIN-MAE
ERIN-MAI
ERIN-MARIE
ERIN-MAY
ERIN-ROSE
ERINA
ERIND
ERINE
ERINN
ERINNA
ERINNE
ERINOLUWA
ERIOLUWA
ERION
ERIS
ERISA
ERISELDA
ERJON
ERJONA
ERKAN
ERLA
ERLANDAS
ERLIS
ERLISA
ERMAL
ERMAN
ERMELA
ERMIAS
ERMINA
ERMIR
ERMIRA
ERMIS
ERNA
ERNEST
ERNESTAS
ERNESTINA
ERNESTINE
ERNESTO
ERNESTS
ERNIE
ERNIS
EROL
EROMOSELE
ERON
ERONA
EROS
ERRAN
ERRIN
ERRIS
ERROL
ERROLL
ERRON
ERRYN
ERSA
ERSAN
ERSIN
ERTAN
ERTUGRUL
ERUM
ERVA
ERVIN
ERVINAS
ERVIS
ERWAN
ERWIN
ERYK
ERYKA
ERYKAH
ERYL
ERYN
ERYNN
ERYS
ERZA
ESA
ESAA
ESAAH
ESAAM
ESAH
ESAM
ESAMAE
ESAMAI
ESDRAS
ESE
ESELD
ESEN
ESENGUL
ESEOGHENE
ESEOSA
ESER
ESEY
ESHA
ESHAA
ESHAAL
ESHAAN
ESHAANI
ESHAH
ESHAL
ESHAN
ESHANA
ESHANI
ESHAR
ESHE
ESHER
ESHIKA
ESHITA
ESHWAR
ESI
ESILA
ESIN
ESINAM
ESKIL
ESKILD
ESLEM
ESMA
ESMAE
ESMAE-GRACE
ESMAE-LOUISE
ESMAE-ROSE
ESMAI
ESMAI-ROSE
ESMAII
ESMAIL
ESMANUR
ESMAY
ESME
ESME-GRACE
ESME-JADE
ESME-LOUISE
ESME-MARIE
ESME-RAE
ESME-ROSE
ESMEA
ESMEE
ESMEE-LOUISE
ESMEE-ROSE
ESMERALDA
ESMERELDA
ESMI

ESMIA	ETHAN-DANIEL	EVA-MAE
ESMIE	ETHAN-JACK	EVA-MAI
ESMIRA	ETHAN-JAMES	EVA-MARIA
ESMOND	ETHAN-JAY	EVA-MARIE
ESOHE	ETHAN-JOHN	EVA-MAY
ESOSA	ETHAN-LEE	EVA-RAE
ESPEN	ETHAN-THOMAS	EVA-ROSE
ESPERANCE	ETHANIEL	EVA-SOPHIA
ESPERANZA	ETHEL	EVAAN
ESRA	ETHEM	EVAH
ESRAA	ETHEN	EVALEIGH
ESROM	ETHIAN	EVALIE
ESSA	ETHNE	EVALIN
ESSAH	ETHNI	EVALINA
ESSAM	ETHOLLE	EVALINE
ESSAN	ETHYN	EVALYN
ESSENCE	ETIEN	EVALYNE
ESSEY	ETIENNE	EVALYNN
ESSI	ETINOSA	EVALYNNE
ESSIA	ETOILE	EVAN
ESSIE	ETTA	EVANA
ESSIEN	ETTA-MAE	EVANAH
ESTA	ETTIE	EVANAS
ESTEBAN	ETTIENNE	EVANDER
ESTEE	ETTORE	EVANGALINE
ESTELA	ETTY	EVANGELENE
ESTELLA	EUAN	EVANGELIA
ESTELLE	EUDORA	EVANGELINA
ESTER	EUGEN	EVANGELINE
ESTERA	EUGENE	EVANGELOS
ESTERE	EUGENIA	EVANI
ESTHER	EUGENIE	EVANIA
ESTHER-ROSE	EUGENIO	EVANN
ESTI	EULALIA	EVANNA
ESTON	EULALIE	EVANNAH
ESTRA	EUN	EVANNE
ESTRELA	EUNICE	EVANS
ESTRELLA	EUPHEMIA	EVANTHE
ESTY	EURON	EVANTHIA
ESTYN	EUROS	EVAYA
ESYLLT	EVA	EVE
ESZTER	EVA-BELLE	EVEA
ETAIN	EVA-GRACE	EVEE
ETAN	EVA-JANE	EVEIE
ETANA	EVA-JEAN	EVELEEN
ETANAS	EVA-LEIGH	EVELEIGH
ETERNITY	EVA-LILY	EVELIA
ETHAN	EVA-LOUISE	EVELIEN

EVELIN
EVELINA
EVELINE
EVELLYN
EVELYN
EVELYN-GRACE
EVELYN-MAE
EVELYN-MAY
EVELYN-ROSE
EVELYNA
EVELYNE
EVELYNN
EVELYNN-ROSE
EVELYNNE
EVEN
EVER
EVEREST
EVERETT
EVERLEIGH
EVERLEY
EVERLIE
EVERLY
EVERLYN
EVERLYNN
EVERSON
EVERT
EVERTON
EVETTE
EVEY
EVI
EVIA
EVIANA
EVIE
EVIE-
EVIE-ANN
EVIE-ANNE
EVIE-BELLE
EVIE-BLOSSOM
EVIE-ELIZABETH
EVIE-FAITH
EVIE-GRACE
EVIE-HOPE
EVIE-JADE
EVIE-JAE
EVIE-JAI
EVIE-JANE
EVIE-JAYNE
EVIE-JEAN
EVIE-JO
EVIE-LEA
EVIE-LEE
EVIE-LEIGH
EVIE-LILLY
EVIE-LOU
EVIE-LOUISE
EVIE-LYNN
EVIE-MAE
EVIE-MAI
EVIE-MARIA
EVIE-MARIE
EVIE-MAY
EVIE-RAE
EVIE-ROSE
EVIE-SUE
EVIE-WILLOW
EVIEE
EVIIE
EVIJA
EVIN
EVINA
EVISSA
EVITA
EVLIN
EVLYN
EVLYNN
EVNI
EVOLET
EVON
EVONY
EVREN
EVRON
EVVIE
EVY
EVYN
EWA
EWAN
EWAOLUWA
EWART
EWELINA
EWEN
EWOMAZINO
EWURA
EWYN
EXAUCE
EXAUCEE
EXCEL
EXCELLENCE
EXCELLENT
EXODUS
EYAD
EYAL
EYAS
EYDIE
EYHAB
EYITAYO
EYLA
EYLEM
EYLUL
EYMAN
EYMEN
EYOB
EYOEL
EYRA
EYRAH
EYSAN
EYSHA
EYTAN
EYTHAN
EYUB
EYUP
EYVA
EZAAN
EZAN
EZANA
EZARA
EZECHIEL
EZEKIEL
EZEL
EZEQUIEL
EZGI
EZINNE
EZIO
EZMAE
EZMAE-ROSE
EZMAI
EZMAY
EZME
EZMEE
EZMIE
EZMIRA
EZO
EZRA
EZRA-JAMES
EZRAE

EZRAH
EZRI
EZRIEL
EZZAH

F

FAA'IZAH
FAAIZ
FAAIZA
FAAIZAH
FAAKHIR
FAARIA
FAARIHA
FAARIS
FAATIMA
FAATIMA-ZAHRA
FAATIMAH
FAAZ
FABBIHA
FABEHA
FABIA
FABIAN
FABIANA
FABIANO
FABIEN
FABIENNE
FABIHA
FABIO
FABIOLA
FABION
FABLE
FABLIHA
FABRICE
FABRICIO
FABRIZIO
FADEELAH
FADEL
FADHIL
FADI
FADIA
FADIL
FADILA
FADIMA
FADIME
FADUMA
FADUMO
FADWA
FADZAI
FAE
FAEEZA

FAELAN
FAEZA
FAEZAH
FAFA
FAHAD
FAHD
FAHED
FAHEEM
FAHEEMA
FAHEEMAH
FAHEMA
FAHID
FAHIM
FAHIMA
FAHIMAH
FAHIMUL
FAHIZA
FAHMEDA
FAHMI
FAHMID
FAHMIDA
FAHMIDAH
FAHMINA
FAHREN
FAHRIN
FAHTIMA
FAI
FAIGA
FAIGE
FAIGY
FAIHA
FAIMA
FAIQ
FAIQA
FAISA
FAISAL
FAISEL
FAITH
FAITH-LOUISE
FAITH-MARIE
FAITH-ROSE
FAITHE
FAITHIA
FAIYAZ
FAIZ
FAIZA
FAIZAAN
FAIZAH

FAIZAL
FAIZAN
FAJAR
FAJER
FAJR
FAKHIR
FALAK
FALAN
FALAQ
FALEN
FALIHA
FALISHA
FALLON
FALLOU
FALLYN
FALON
FAMKE
FANE
FANTA
FANTASIA
FANUEL
FAOLAN
FARA
FARAAZ
FARADAY
FARAH
FARAI
FARAJ
FARAN
FARAZ
FARDEEN
FARDIN
FARDOSA
FARDOWSA
FAREED
FAREEDA
FAREEDAH
FAREEDAT
FAREEHA
FAREEN
FAREENA
FAREES
FAREHA
FAREN
FARES
FARHA
FARHAAD
FARHAAN

FARHAD
FARHAN
FARHANA
FARHANAH
FARHAT
FARHEEN
FARHIA
FARHIN
FARHIYA
FARIA
FARIAH
FARID
FARIDA
FARIDAH
FARIDAT
FARIDEH
FARIHA
FARIHAH
FARINA
FARIS
FARISHA
FARIYA
FARIYAH
FARIZ
FARJANA
FARKHAN
FARLEY
FARMAN
FARNAZ
FARON
FAROOQ
FAROUK
FAROUQ
FARRADEH
FARRAH
FARRAN
FARREL
FARRELL
FARREN
FARRIN
FARRIS
FARRON
FARRUKH
FARRYL
FARRYN
FARTUN
FARUK
FARUQ
FARWA
FARWAH
FARYAAL
FARYAL
FARYL
FARYN
FARZAD
FARZAN
FARZANA
FARZEEN
FASEEH
FASEEHA
FASIHA
FATAMA
FATEEMA
FATEH
FATEHA
FATEMA
FATEMAH
FATEMEH
FATHEHA
FATHEMA
FATHIA
FATHIMA
FATHIMAH
FATHIYA
FATHMA
FATIH
FATIHA
FATIHAH
FATIM
FATIMA
FATIMA-TUZ-ZAHRA
FATIMA-ZAHRA
FATIMAH
FATIMAH-ZAHRA
FATIMAH-ZAHRAH
FATIMAHZAHRA
FATIMAT
FATIMATOU
FATIN
FATMA
FATMAH
FATMANUR
FATMATA
FATOS
FATOU
FATOUMATA
FATOUMATTA
FATUMA
FATUMATA
FAUNA
FAUSTA
FAUSTAS
FAUSTE
FAUSTINA
FAUSTINE
FAUSTO
FAUSTYNA
FAUVE
FAUZAN
FAUZIA
FAUZIAH
FAVOR
FAVOUR
FAWAAZ
FAWAD
FAWAZ
FAWN
FAWWAZ
FAWZAAN
FAWZAN
FAWZIA
FAWZIYA
FAWZIYAH
FAY
FAYA
FAYAAZ
FAYAZ
FAYE
FAYE-LOUISE
FAYE-MARIE
FAYED
FAYEZ
FAYHA
FAYOLA
FAYROUZ
FAYSAL
FAYTH
FAYTHE
FAYYAD
FAYYAZ
FAYZA
FAYZAAN
FAYZAN
FAZAAN

FAZAL
FAZAN
FAZEEL
FAZEELA
FAZER
FAZIL
FAZILA
FEARGHAL
FEARGHUS
FEARGUS
FEARN
FEARNE
FEBA
FEBE
FEBIN
FEDERICA
FEDERICO
FEDOR
FEDORA
FEHZAAN
FEHZAN
FEI
FEIGE
FEIGY
FEISAL
FEIVEL
FELESHA
FELICE
FELICIA
FELICITAS
FELICITE
FELICITY
FELICITY-MAY
FELICITY-ROSE
FELICJA
FELIKS
FELIPE
FELISHA
FELIX
FEMI
FEMKE
FEN
FENELLA
FENIL
FENIX
FENN
FENNA
FENNELLA

FENNER
FENTON
FEODOR
FERAH
FERAS
FERDAWS
FERDIA
FERDIE
FERDINAND
FERDOUS
FERDOUSI
FERDOWS
FERENC
FERGAL
FERGUS
FERGUSON
FERHAN
FERHAT
FERIDE
FERIEL
FERN
FERNANDA
FERNANDO
FERNE
FERNLEY
FERON
FEROZ
FEROZE
FERRAN
FERRELL
FERRIS
FESTUS
FEVEN
FEYISAYO
FEYNMAN
FEYSAL
FEYZA
FEZA
FEZAAN
FEZAN
FEZHAN
FFION
FFLUR
FFYON
FFYONA
FIA
FIACHRA
FIADH

FIAMMA
FIANNA
FIAZ
FIAZA
FIDA
FIDAH
FIDAN
FIDEL
FIDELIS
FIFI
FIIFI
FIKRET
FILIP
FILIPA
FILIPE
FILIPP
FILIPPA
FILIPPO
FILIPPOS
FILIPS
FILIZ
FILLIP
FILMON
FILSAN
FILZA
FIN
FINA
FINAN
FINBAR
FINBARR
FINCH
FINDLAY
FINDLEY
FINEAS
FINELLA
FINIAN
FINJA
FINLAE
FINLAN
FINLAY
FINLEA
FINLEE
FINLEIGH
FINLEY
FINLEY-J
FINLEY-JAMES
FINLEY-JAY
FINLO

FINLY	FIZAA	FLYNT
FINN	FIZAAN	FODAY
FINNAN	FIZAH	FOLABOMI
FINNBAR	FIZAN	FOLAKE
FINNBARR	FIZZA	FOLAKEMI
FINNEGAN	FIZZAH	FOLARIN
FINNEN	FJOLLA	FOLASADE
FINNIAN	FLAVIA	FOLASHADE
FINNICK	FLAVIAN	FORBES
FINNIGAN	FLAVIO	FORD
FINNLAY	FLAVIUS	FOREST
FINNLEA	FLETCHER	FORHAD
FINNLEE	FLEUR	FORID
FINNLEIGH	FLINN	FORIDA
FINNLEY	FLINT	FORREST
FINNLY	FLO	FORTUNA
FINNTAN	FLOELLA	FORTUNE
FINOLA	FLORA	FOSTER
FINTAN	FLORANCE	FOUAD
FINTON	FLOREN	FOUZIA
FINTY	FLORENA	FOWZIA
FION	FLORENCE	FOX
FIONA	FLORENCE-MAY	FOXX
FIONN	FLORENCE-ROSE	FOY
FIONNA	FLORENCIA	FOYEZ
FIONNAN	FLORENT	FOYZUL
FIONNLAGH	FLORENTIA	FOZIA
FIONNOULA	FLORENTINA	FRADEL
FIONNTAN	FLORENTINE	FRAIDA
FIONNUALA	FLORES	FRAISER
FIONNULA	FLORI	FRAIYA
FIORELLA	FLORIA	FRAIZER
FIRAS	FLORIAN	FRAN
FIRAT	FLORIANA	FRANCA
FIRAZ	FLORIANE	FRANCES
FIRDAUS	FLORIE	FRANCESCA
FIRDAWS	FLORIN	FRANCESCA-ROSE
FIRDOUS	FLORINA	FRANCESCO
FIRDOWS	FLORIS	FRANCESKA
FIROZA	FLORJAN	FRANCESSCA
FISHER	FLORRIE	FRANCHESCA
FISNIK	FLORYN	FRANCHESKA
FITCH	FLOSSIE	FRANCIE
FITZGERALD	FLOSSY	FRANCINE
FITZROY	FLOURISH	FRANCIS
FIYINFOLUWA	FLOYD	FRANCISCA
FIYINFUNOLUWA	FLYN	FRANCISCO
FIZA	FLYNN	FRANCISZEK

FRANCISZKA
FRANCK
FRANCO
FRANCOIS
FRANCOISE
FRANEK
FRANK
FRANKA
FRANKE
FRANKEE
FRANKEY
FRANKI
FRANKIE
FRANKIE-ANN
FRANKIE-DEAN
FRANKIE-GEORGE
FRANKIE-J
FRANKIE-JAMES
FRANKIE-JANE
FRANKIE-JAY
FRANKIE-JO
FRANKIE-JOE
FRANKIE-JOHN
FRANKIE-LEA
FRANKIE-LEE
FRANKIE-LEIGH
FRANKIE-LOU
FRANKIE-LOUISE
FRANKIE-MAE
FRANKIE-MAI
FRANKIE-MARIE
FRANKIE-MAY
FRANKIE-RAE
FRANKIE-RAY
FRANKIE-ROSE
FRANKIEE
FRANKII
FRANKLIN
FRANKLYN
FRANKO
FRANKY
FRANTISEK
FRANZ
FRANZISKA
FRASER
FRASIER
FRAYA
FRAYAH

FRAYER
FRAZ
FRAZER
FRAZEY
FRAZIER
FREA
FRED
FREDA
FREDDI
FREDDIE
FREDDIE-DEAN
FREDDIE-GEORGE
FREDDIE-JAMES
FREDDIE-JAY
FREDDIE-JOE
FREDDIE-JOHN
FREDDIE-LEE
FREDDIE-RAY
FREDDY
FREDDY-GEORGE
FREDDY-JAMES
FREDDY-LEE
FREDERIC
FREDERICA
FREDERICK
FREDERICO
FREDERIK
FREDERIKA
FREDERIQUE
FREDI
FREDRIC
FREDRICK
FREDRIK
FREDRIKA
FREEDA
FREEDOM
FREEMAN
FREIA
FREIDA
FREIDY
FREIJA
FREIYA
FREJA
FRENCHIE
FRESHTA
FREY
FREYA
FREYA-ANN

FREYA-ANNE
FREYA-GRACE
FREYA-LEIGH
FREYA-LILLY
FREYA-LILY
FREYA-LOUISE
FREYA-MAE
FREYA-MAI
FREYA-MARIE
FREYA-MAY
FREYA-ROSE
FREYAH
FREYIA
FREYJA
FREYJA-ROSE
FRIDA
FRIEDA
FRIEDERIKE
FRIEDRICH
FRIEDY
FRIMET
FRISHTA
FRITZ
FRUZSINA
FRYDERYK
FUAAD
FUAD
FUCHSIA
FUNMILAYO
FUNMILOLA
FURKAN
FURQAAN
FURQAN
FUZAIL
FYFE
FYN
FYNLAY
FYNLEE
FYNLEY
FYNN
FYNNLAY
FYNNLEY
FYNTON
FYODOR
FYZA

G

GABBIE
GABBY
GABE
GABI
GABIA
GABIJA
GABIN
GABOR
GABRIAL
GABRIAN
GABRIEL
GABRIELA
GABRIELE
GABRIELIS
GABRIELIUS
GABRIELLA
GABRIELLA-ROSE
GABRIELLE
GABRIELS
GABY
GAD
GADI
GADIEL
GAEL
GAELEN
GAELLE
GAETAN
GAETANO
GAGAN
GAGANDEEP
GAGANPREET
GAGE
GAIA
GAIGE
GAIL
GAIUS
GAIZKA
GAJA
GAL
GALA
GALEN
GALENA
GALIA
GALILEO
GALINA
GALLA
GALLAGHER
GALVIN
GAMAL
GAMAR
GAMZE
GANESH
GANEVE
GANGA
GAR
GARAN
GARANCE
GARETH
GARGI
GARIMA
GARIN
GARION
GARMON
GARON
GARREN
GARRET
GARRETH
GARRETT
GARRICK
GARRISON
GARRY
GARTH
GARV
GARVEY
GARY
GARYN
GASPAR
GASPARD
GASTON
GAURAV
GAURI
GAURIKA
GAUTAM
GAUTHAM
GAVAN
GAVIN
GAVINDEEP
GAVINDER
GAVRIEL
GAVRIELLA
GAVYN
GAWAIN
GAY
GAYA
GAYATHIRI
GAYATHRI
GAYATRI
GAYLE
GAYNOR
GAZEL
GAZI
GBEMISOLA
GBOLAHAN
GEAROID
GED
GEDALIA
GEDALYA
GEDEON
GEDIMINAS
GEENA
GEET
GEETA
GEETIKA
GELILA
GEM
GEMIMA
GEMINI
GEMMA
GEMMA-LOUISE
GENA
GENE
GENESIS
GENEVA
GENEVE
GENEVIEVE
GENEZA
GENIE
GENNA
GENNARO
GENO
GENSON
GENT
GENTA
GENTIAN
GENTIANA
GENTRIT
GEO
GEOFF
GEOFFREY
GEORDAN

GEORDIE
GEORG
GEORGA
GEORGE
GEORGE-HENRY
GEORGE-JAMES
GEORGE-WILLIAM
GEORGEA
GEORGEANA
GEORGEE
GEORGEINA
GEORGENA
GEORGES
GEORGETTE
GEORGEY
GEORGI
GEORGIA
GEORGIA-GRACE
GEORGIA-LEE
GEORGIA-LEIGH
GEORGIA-LOUISE
GEORGIA-MAE
GEORGIA-MAI
GEORGIA-MAY
GEORGIA-RAE
GEORGIA-ROSE
GEORGIANA
GEORGIANNA
GEORGIE
GEORGIE-ANN
GEORGIE-LEE
GEORGIE-LEIGH
GEORGIE-MAE
GEORGIE-MAI
GEORGIE-MAY
GEORGIE-RAE
GEORGIE-ROSE
GEORGINA
GEORGINA-ROSE
GEORGIO
GEORGIOS
GEORGIY
GEORGY
GEORJA
GEOVANNA
GEOVANNI
GERAINT
GERALD

GERALDINE
GERALLT
GERARD
GERARDAS
GERASIMOS
GERDA
GERGANA
GERGELY
GERGO
GERI
GERMAIN
GERMAINE
GEROME
GERONIMO
GERRAN
GERRARD
GERRI
GERRY
GERSHON
GERSON
GERTA
GERTIE
GERTRUDE
GERVAIS
GERWYN
GESSICA
GETHEN
GETHIN
GETHYN
GEVORG
GEZIM
GHADA
GHADEER
GHAFOOR
GHALA
GHALIB
GHANIA
GHANIM
GHASSAN
GHAZAL
GHAZALA
GHAZI
GHENA
GHEORGHE
GHINA
GHISLAINE
GHITA
GHULAM

GHYLL
GIA
GIAAN
GIACOMO
GIADA
GIAN
GIAN-LUCA
GIANA
GIANCARLO
GIANFRANCO
GIANLUCA
GIANLUCCA
GIANMARCO
GIANNA
GIANNI
GIANNIS
GIANPAOLO
GIAVANNA
GIBRAN
GIBRIL
GIBSON
GIDEON
GIDON
GIFT
GIFTY
GIGI
GIHAN
GIL
GILA
GILAD
GILBERT
GILBY
GILDA
GILEAD
GILES
GILLAN
GILLEN
GILLES
GILLESPIE
GILLIAN
GILLY
GINA
GINEVRA
GINIKA
GINNIE
GINNY
GINO
GINTARE

GIO
GIOELE
GIOIA
GIORDANO
GIORGI
GIORGIA
GIORGIANA
GIORGINA
GIORGIO
GIOVANI
GIOVANNA
GIOVANNI
GIOVANNY
GIPSY
GIRAY
GIRISH
GISELA
GISELE
GISELLA
GISELLE
GITA
GITEL
GITTEL
GITTY
GIULIA
GIULIANA
GIULIANO
GIULIETTA
GIULIO
GIUSEPPE
GIUSEPPINA
GIVEN
GIVERNY
GIYA
GIZELLE
GIZEM
GJERGJ
GLADWIN
GLADYS
GLAIN
GLEB
GLEN
GLENA
GLENDA
GLENDON
GLENN
GLESNI
GLODI
GLODY
GLORIA
GLORIANA
GLORIJA
GLORIOUS
GLORY
GLYN
GLYNN
GOBIND
GODA
GODFRED
GODFREY
GODIVA
GODRIC
GODSON
GODSWILL
GODWILL
GODWIN
GOHAR
GOKAY
GOKCE
GOKDENIZ
GOKHAN
GOKUL
GOKULAN
GOLAM
GOLDA
GOLDEN
GOLDIE
GOLDY
GONCALO
GONUL
GONZALO
GOODLUCK
GOODNESS
GOPAL
GOPIKA
GORAN
GORDON
GORGIA
GORKEM
GOSPEL
GOURAV
GOURI
GOUTHAM
GOVIND
GOVINDER
GOWRI
GOWTHAM
GOZDE
GRACE
GRACE-ELIZABETH
GRACE-KELLY
GRACE-LEIGH
GRACE-LILY
GRACE-LOUISE
GRACE-MARIE
GRACE-MAY
GRACE-OLIVIA
GRACE-ROSE
GRACEE
GRACELYN
GRACEY
GRACEY-MAI
GRACEY-MAY
GRACI
GRACIA
GRACIAN
GRACIANA
GRACIE
GRACIE-
GRACIE-ANN
GRACIE-ANNE
GRACIE-BELLE
GRACIE-ELLA
GRACIE-JANE
GRACIE-JAYNE
GRACIE-JEAN
GRACIE-JO
GRACIE-LEA
GRACIE-LEE
GRACIE-LEIGH
GRACIE-LOU
GRACIE-LOUISE
GRACIE-MAE
GRACIE-MAI
GRACIE-MARIE
GRACIE-MAY
GRACIE-RAE
GRACIE-ROSE
GRACIELA
GRACIELLA
GRACIEMAY
GRACIENNE
GRACIOUS
GRACJAN

GRACY
GRADI
GRADY
GRAE
GRAEME
GRAHAM
GRAHAME
GRAICE
GRAINNE
GRANIA
GRANIT
GRANT
GRANTAS
GRAY
GRAYCE
GRAYCIE
GRAYDON
GRAYSEN
GRAYSON
GRAZIA
GRAZIELLA
GREAT
GREATNESS
GREER
GREG
GREGG
GREGOIRE
GREGOR
GREGORIO
GREGORY
GREIG
GREISI
GREJSI
GRESA
GRETA
GRETCHEN
GRETEL
GRETTA
GREY
GREYSEN
GREYSON
GRIFF
GRIFFIN
GRIFFITH
GRIFFYDD
GRIFFYN
GRIGORIOS
GRIGORIY

GRISELDA
GRISHMA
GRISMA
GRUFF
GRUFFUDD
GRUFFYDD
GRYFF
GRYFFIN
GRZEGORZ
GUGANDEEP
GUGLIELMO
GUIDO
GUILHERME
GUILLAUME
GUILLERMO
GUINEVERE
GUISEPPE
GUL
GULAM
GULAY
GULCAN
GULCIN
GULED
GULEED
GULEID
GULIZAR
GULLIVER
GULLU
GULRAIZ
GULSAH
GULSEN
GULSHAN
GULSUM
GULUSTAN
GULUZAR
GUNAY
GUNEET
GUNES
GUNEY
GUNNAR
GUNNER
GUNREET
GUNVEER
GURAMRIT
GURANSH
GURASEES
GURBANI
GURBIR

GURCHARAN
GURCHETAN
GURDAS
GURDEEP
GURDEV
GURDIT
GUREKAM
GURFATEH
GURINDER
GURJAS
GURJEET
GURJEEVAN
GURJINDER
GURJIT
GURJOT
GURJYOT
GURKAMAL
GURKAN
GURKARAN
GURKIRAN
GURKIRAT
GURLEEN
GURMAAN
GURMAN
GURMEET
GURMINDER
GURMUKH
GURNAAZ
GURNAIK
GURNAM
GURNEET
GURNEK
GURNOOR
GURPAL
GURPARTAP
GURPREET
GURPRIYA
GURRAJ
GURREET
GURSAHEJ
GURSAHIB
GURSEERAT
GURSEHAJ
GURSEV
GURSEVAK
GURSEWAK
GURSHAAN
GURSHAN

GURSHARAN
GURSHARON
GURSIMAR
GURSIMRAN
GURSIRAT
GURTAAJ
GURTAJ
GURTARAN
GURTEJ
GURVEEN
GURVEER
GURVINDER
GURVIR
GUS
GUSTAF
GUSTAS
GUSTAV
GUSTAVE
GUSTAVO
GUSTAVS
GUSTAW
GUSTE
GUTO
GUVEN
GUY
GVIDAS
GWAWR
GWEN
GWENAN
GWENDOLEN
GWENDOLINE
GWENDOLYN
GWENETH
GWENEVERE
GWENI
GWENLLI
GWENLLIAN
GWENNA
GWENNAN
GWENNIE
GWENNO
GWENO
GWENYTH
GWERN
GWILYM
GWION
GWYDION
GWYN
GWYNDAF
GWYNETH
GWYNFOR
GYAAN
GYAN
GYLES
GYORGY
GYPSEY
GYPSIE
GYPSY
GYPSY-MAY
GYPSY-ROSE
GYTIS

H

H	HABIIBA	HADY
HA	HABIL	HADYA
HAAD	HABON	HADYN
HAADI	HABOON	HAF
HAADIA	HACI	HAFEEZ
HAADIYA	HADAR	HAFEEZA
HAADIYAH	HADARA	HAFEEZAH
HAAFIZAH	HADASA	HAFEZA
HAAJAR	HADASSA	HAFINA
HAAJARAH	HADASSAH	HAFIZ
HAAJIRA	HADDEN	HAFIZA
HAAJIRAH	HADDIE	HAFIZAH
HAAJRA	HADDIJATOU	HAFIZUR
HAAJRAH	HADDON	HAFSA
HAALA	HADDY	HAFSAH
HAALAH	HADDYJATOU	HAFSAT
HAAMID	HADEAL	HAFSHA
HAANA	HADEE	HAFSO
HAANI	HADEED	HAFSSA
HAANIA	HADEEL	HAFWEN
HAANIAH	HADEEQA	HAFZA
HAANIYA	HADEEQAH	HAFZAH
HAANIYAH	HADEN	HAGAN
HAARIS	HADER	HAGEN
HAARISAH	HADI	HAGER
HAARITH	HADIA	HAI
HAAROON	HADIAH	HAIDAN
HAASHIM	HADID	HAIDAR
HAASHIR	HADIJA	HAIDEE
HAASINI	HADIJATOU	HAIDEN
HAAWA	HADIKA	HAIDER
HAAZIQ	HADIL	HAIDER-ALI
HABEEB	HADIQA	HAIDON
HABEEBA	HADIQAH	HAIDYN
HABEEBAH	HADIS	HAIFA
HABEEL	HADIYA	HAIG
HABEN	HADIYAH	HAIKA
HABIB	HADIYYAH	HAIKAL
HABIBA	HADIZA	HAILA
HABIBAH	HADJA	HAILE
HABIBAT	HADJER	HAILEE
HABIBUL	HADLEE	HAILEY
HABIBULLAH	HADLEIGH	HAILIE
HABIBUR	HADLEY	HAILIE-JADE
	HADLEY-JAMES	HAILLIE
	HADRIAN	HAIMI
	HADRIEL	HAIQA
	HADRIEN	HAIQAH

HAISAM	HALINA	HAMIDULLAH
HAITHAM	HALIT	HAMILTON
HAITHEM	HALIYAH	HAMIM
HAIZEA	HALIYAT	HAMIMA
HAJA	HALLA	HAMISH
HAJAR	HALLAM	HAMIZ
HAJARA	HALLE	HAMMAAD
HAJARAH	HALLE-MAE	HAMMAD
HAJER	HALLE-MAI	HAMMAM
HAJERA	HALLE-MAY	HAMMED
HAJERAH	HALLE-RAE	HAMNA
HAJIR	HALLE-ROSE	HAMNAH
HAJIRA	HALLEE	HAMOOD
HAJIRAH	HALLEY	HAMSA
HAJR	HALLI	HAMSE
HAJRA	HALLIE	HAMZA
HAJRAH	HALLIE-GRACE	HAMZAH
HAKAN	HALLIE-MAE	HAMZE
HAKEEM	HALLIE-MAI	HAN
HAKIM	HALLIE-MARIE	HANA
HAKIMA	HALLIE-MAY	HANAA
HAL	HALLIE-RAE	HANAAN
HALA	HALLIE-ROSE	HANAD
HALAH	HALLUM	HANADI
HALAINA	HALLY	HANAE
HALDEN	HALO	HANAH
HALE	HAMAAD	HANAIYA
HALEEM	HAMAD	HANAKO
HALEEMA	HAMAS	HANAN
HALEEMA-SADIA	HAMASA	HANAR
HALEEMAH	HAMAZ	HANASA
HALEEMAT	HAMD	HANAYA
HALEENA	HAMDA	HANEEF
HALEIGH	HAMDAAN	HANEEFA
HALEMA	HAMDAH	HANEEFAH
HALEN	HAMDAN	HANEEN
HALENA	HAMDI	HANEET
HALEY	HAMDY	HANFA
HALI	HAMED	HANFAA
HALIA	HAMEDA	HANG
HALIE	HAMEED	HANGA
HALIL	HAMEEDA	HANI
HALIM	HAMEEDAH	HANIA
HALIMA	HAMEEM	HANIAH
HALIMA-SADIA	HAMERA	HANIEH
HALIMAH	HAMID	HANIEL
HALIMAT	HAMIDA	HANIF
HALIMO	HAMIDAH	HANIFA

HANIFAH	HANZALAH	HARIT
HANIFE	HANZLAH	HARITA
HANIKA	HAO	HARITH
HANIN	HAORAN	HARITHA
HANISH	HAOXUAN	HARIZ
HANISHA	HAOYU	HARJAAP
HANIYA	HAPPINESS	HARJAN
HANIYAH	HAQEEM	HARJAP
HANIYYA	HARAJAN	HARJAS
HANIYYAH	HARALAMBOS	HARJEET
HANK	HARALD	HARJEEVAN
HANLEY	HARAM	HARJINDER
HANLON	HARAN	HARJIT
HANNA	HARAS	HARJIVAN
HANNAA	HARBINDER	HARJODH
HANNAH	HARBIR	HARJOT
HANNAH-GRACE	HARBOR	HARJOTH
HANNAH-JAYNE	HARBOUR	HARJOVAN
HANNAH-LEIGH	HARDEEP	HARJUN
HANNAH-LOUISE	HARDEV	HARJYOT
HANNAH-MAE	HARDIK	HARKARAN
HANNAH-MARIE	HARDIT	HARKEERAT
HANNAH-MAY	HARDY	HARKIERAN
HANNAH-ROSE	HAREEM	HARKIRAN
HANNALISE	HAREENA	HARKIRAT
HANNAN	HAREER	HARKRISHAN
HANNE	HAREES	HARLA
HANNELORE	HAREL	HARLAN
HANNES	HARESH	HARLAND
HANNI	HARETH	HARLEA
HANNIBAL	HARFATEH	HARLEE
HANNIEL	HARGUN	HARLEE-MAE
HANNIYA	HARI	HARLEEN
HANNO	HARIETTE	HARLEI
HANO	HARIHARAN	HARLEIGH
HANS	HARIN	HARLEIGH-MAE
HANSA	HARINDER	HARLEIGH-MAI
HANSAH	HARINE	HARLEIGH-RAE
HANSEL	HARINI	HARLEM
HANSEN	HARIS	HARLEN
HANSHIKA	HARISA	HARLEY
HANSIKA	HARISAH	HARLEY-DEAN
HANSINI	HARISAN	HARLEY-J
HANSON	HARISH	HARLEY-JACK
HANY	HARISHAN	HARLEY-JAE
HANYA	HARISON	HARLEY-JAI
HANZ	HARISS	HARLEY-JAMES
HANZALA	HARISSON	HARLEY-JAY

HARLEY-JOE
HARLEY-JOHN
HARLEY-LEE
HARLEY-MAE
HARLEY-MAY
HARLEY-OWEN
HARLEY-QUINN
HARLEY-RAE
HARLEY-RAY
HARLEY-REECE
HARLEY-ROSE
HARLI
HARLIE
HARLIE-GRACE
HARLIE-RAE
HARLIE-ROSE
HARLIN
HARLO
HARLOE
HARLOW
HARLOW-ROSE
HARLOWE
HARLUN
HARLY
HARLYN
HARMAAN
HARMAN
HARMANDEEP
HARMANI
HARMANJIT
HARMANNAT
HARMANPREET
HARMEET
HARMINDER
HARMONEY
HARMONI
HARMONIE
HARMONIE-ROSE
HARMONY
HARMONY-GRACE
HARMONY-ROSE
HARNAIK
HARNAM
HARNEET
HARNEK
HARNOOP
HARNOOR
HAROLD

HAROLDAS
HARON
HAROON
HAROUN
HARPA
HARPAL
HARPER
HARPER-GRACE
HARPER-JANE
HARPER-JEAN
HARPER-JO
HARPER-LEA
HARPER-LEE
HARPER-LEIGH
HARPER-LILLIE
HARPER-LILLY
HARPER-LILY
HARPER-LOUISE
HARPER-MAE
HARPER-MAI
HARPER-MAY
HARPER-RAE
HARPER-ROSE
HARPER-WILLOW
HARPREET
HARPRIYA
HARRAJ
HARRI
HARRIE
HARRIET
HARRIET-ROSE
HARRIETT
HARRIETTA
HARRIETTE
HARRINGTON
HARRIOT
HARRIOTT
HARRIS
HARRISEN
HARRISH
HARRISON
HARRISON-BLAKE
HARRISON-JAMES
HARRISON-LEE
HARRISSON
HARROOP
HARRY
HARRY-DAVID

HARRY-GEORGE
HARRY-JACK
HARRY-JAMES
HARRY-JAY
HARRY-JOE
HARRY-JOHN
HARRY-LEE
HARRYSON
HARSAHIB
HARSEERAT
HARSH
HARSHA
HARSHAAN
HARSHAL
HARSHAN
HARSHARAN
HARSHDEEP
HARSHI
HARSHIKA
HARSHIL
HARSHINI
HARSHITA
HARSHITH
HARSHITHA
HARSHIV
HARSHNI
HARSHVEER
HARSIMAR
HARSIMRAN
HARSIMRAT
HARSIRAT
HARSUKH
HART
HARTEJ
HARTLEY
HARU
HARUKA
HARUKI
HARUN
HARUNA
HARUTO
HARUUN
HARVEE
HARVEEN
HARVEER
HARVEY
HARVEY-DEAN
HARVEY-GEORGE

88

HARVEY-J	HASINA	HAWDAM
HARVEY-JACK	HASINAH	HAWI
HARVEY-JAI	HASINI	HAWLEY
HARVEY-JAMES	HASNA	HAWRA
HARVEY-JAY	HASNAA	HAWRAA
HARVEY-JOE	HASNAAT	HAWWA
HARVEY-JOHN	HASNAH	HAWWAA
HARVEY-LEE	HASNAIN	HAWWAH
HARVEY-LEIGH	HASNAN	HAWYS
HARVEY-RAY	HASNAT	HAYA
HARVEYLEE	HASNATH	HAYAA
HARVI	HASNAYN	HAYAAN
HARVIE	HASRET	HAYAAT
HARVIN	HASSAAN	HAYAH
HARVIND	HASSAM	HAYAL
HARVINDER	HASSAN	HAYAM
HARVIR	HASSEN	HAYAN
HARVY	HASSNAIN	HAYAT
HARYAD	HASTI	HAYATO
HARYAN	HASTIN	HAYDAN
HASAAM	HASTY	HAYDAR
HASAAN	HASTYAR	HAYDEE
HASAN	HATEM	HAYDEN
HASANA	HATICE	HAYDEN-JAMES
HASANAH	HATIM	HAYDEN-LEE
HASANAIN	HATTI	HAYDER
HASANAT	HATTIE	HAYDN
HASANAYN	HATTIE-MAE	HAYDON
HASEEB	HATTIE-MAY	HAYDYN
HASEEBA	HATTON	HAYES
HASEEBAH	HATTY	HAYET
HASEENA	HAUWA	HAYFA
HASEENAH	HAVA	HAYLA
HASENAT	HAVAL	HAYLEA
HASHAAM	HAVANA	HAYLEE
HASHAM	HAVANAH	HAYLEIGH
HASHEM	HAVANNA	HAYLEN
HASHIM	HAVANNAH	HAYLEY
HASHIR	HAVEN	HAYLEY-JADE
HASHMAT	HAVIN	HAYLEY-JANE
HASHMEET	HAVISH	HAYLEY-MARIE
HASHVEER	HAVISHA	HAYLEY-MAY
HASIB	HAVVA	HAYLIE
HASIBA	HAWA	HAYSAM
HASIBAH	HAWAA	HAYTHAM
HASIFA	HAWABIBI	HAYTHEM
HASIM	HAWAH	HAYWOOD
HASIN	HAWANATU	HAYYA

HAYYAAN	HEIDI-GRACE	HENDERSON
HAYYAN	HEIDI-LEIGH	HENDRICK
HAZAL	HEIDI-LOU	HENDRICKS
HAZAR	HEIDI-MAE	HENDRIK
HAZE	HEIDI-MAY	HENDRIX
HAZEEM	HEIDI-RAE	HENDRY
HAZEL	HEIDI-ROSE	HENG
HAZEL-GRACE	HEINI	HENI
HAZEM	HEINRICH	HENIL
HAZERA	HEITOR	HENLEE
HAZIM	HEJA	HENLEIGH
HAZIQ	HEJAN	HENLEY
HAZIQAH	HEJRAN	HENLEY-JAMES
HAZIRAH	HEKTOR	HENLEY-JOHN
HAZRA	HELA	HENLI
HAZRAT	HELAINA	HENLIE
HE	HELAN	HENLY
HEALEY	HELANA	HENNA
HEATH	HELAYNA	HENNAH
HEATHCLIFF	HELDER	HENNESSEY
HEATHCLIFFE	HELEDD	HENNESSY
HEATHER	HELEENA	HENNIE
HEAVEN	HELEN	HENNING
HEAVEN-LEIGH	HELENA	HENNY
HEAVENLEIGH	HELENE	HENOC
HEAVENLY	HELI	HENOCH
HEAVENLY-JOY	HELIA	HENOCK
HEBA	HELIN	HENOK
HEBAH	HELINA	HENOS
HEBE	HELLA	HENRI
HEBRON	HELLY	HENRICK
HECTOR	HELOISA	HENRIE
HEDAYA	HELOISE	HENRIETTA
HEDD	HEMA	HENRIETTE
HEDDWYN	HEMAL	HENRIJS
HEDI	HEMALI	HENRIK
HEDLEY	HEMAN	HENRIKAS
HEDY	HEMANI	HENRIQUE
HEEBA	HEMANYA	HENRY
HEELA	HEMEN	HENRY-GEORGE
HEENA	HEMI	HENRY-JAMES
HEER	HEMIL	HENRY-JAY
HEERA	HEMISH	HENRY-JOHN
HEERAL	HEMISHA	HENRY-LEE
HEET	HEMMA	HENRY-THOMAS
HEEYA	HENA	HENRYK
HEFIN	HENAL	HENSON
HEIDI	HEND	HEPHZIBAH

HEPZIBAH
HERA
HERAN
HERB
HERBERT
HERBIE
HERCULES
HERKUS
HERMAN
HERMARNI
HERMELA
HERMES
HERMIONE
HERMIONIE
HERMOINE
HERMON
HERO
HERSH
HERSHEL
HERSHI
HERSHY
HERSI
HERVE
HESAM
HESHAM
HESPER
HESSA
HESTER
HESTON
HET
HETAL
HETANSH
HETI
HETTI
HETTIE
HETTIE-MAY
HETTIENNE
HETTY
HETVI
HEULWEN
HEULYN
HEVIN
HEW
HEWAD
HEYABEL
HEYAM
HEYAN
HEYDON

HEZEKIAH
HEZRON
HIBA
HIBAAQ
HIBAH
HIBAQ
HIBATULLAH
HIBBA
HIBBAH
HIBO
HICHAM
HICHEM
HIDAAYAH
HIDAYA
HIDAYAH
HIDEAKI
HIDEO
HIEU
HIFSA
HIFSAH
HIFZA
HIFZAH
HIJAAB
HIJAB
HIJRAH
HIKMA
HIKMAH
HIKMAT
HILA
HILAL
HILARY
HILDA
HILLA
HILLARY
HILLEL
HILMI
HILTON
HIMA
HIMAL
HIMANI
HIMANSHU
HIMAT
HIMESH
HIMMAT
HINA
HINAA
HINAL
HIND

HINDA
HINDI
HINDY
HINESH
HINNA
HIRA
HIRAD
HIRAH
HIRAL
HIRAM
HIRAN
HIRANUR
HIREN
HIRO
HIROKI
HIROKO
HIROTO
HIRRA
HIS
HISHAAM
HISHAM
HISSAN
HITANSH
HITEN
HITESH
HIU
HIVAY
HIVDA
HIYA
HIYAB
HIYABEL
HIYAM
HIZAR
HO
HOA
HOANG
HOBIE
HOCINE
HODA
HODAN
HODO
HODON
HOGAN
HOI
HOK
HOLDEN
HOLI
HOLLAND

HOLLEE	HONEY-MARIE	HRIHAAN
HOLLEIGH	HONEY-MAY	HRISHA
HOLLEY	HONEY-RAE	HRISHI
HOLLI	HONEY-ROSE	HRISHIKESH
HOLLIANNE	HONEYSUCKLE	HRISTO
HOLLIE	HONG	HRITHIK
HOLLIE-ANN	HONI	HRITHIKA
HOLLIE-ANNE	HONIA	HRITIK
HOLLIE-GRACE	HONIE	HRITIKA
HOLLIE-JANE	HONOR	HUBERT
HOLLIE-JO	HONORA	HUBERTAS
HOLLIE-LOUISE	HONORIA	HUCKLEBERRY
HOLLIE-MAE	HONOUR	HUD
HOLLIE-MAI	HONYA	HUDA
HOLLIE-MARIE	HOODA	HUDAA
HOLLIE-MAY	HOODO	HUDAIFA
HOLLIE-RAE	HOOPER	HUDAIFAH
HOLLIE-ROSE	HOOR	HUDAYFA
HOLLIS	HOORAIN	HUDAYFAH
HOLLY	HOORIA	HUDAYFI
HOLLY-	HOORIYA	HUDEYFA
HOLLY-ANN	HOORIYAH	HUDHAIFA
HOLLY-ANNE	HOPE	HUDHAIFAH
HOLLY-GRACE	HOPE-ELIZABETH	HUDHAYFA
HOLLY-JAYNE	HOPE-LOUISE	HUDHAYFAH
HOLLY-JO	HORACE	HUDSON
HOLLY-LOUISE	HORATIO	HUDSON-LEE
HOLLY-MAE	HORIA	HUEY
HOLLY-MAI	HOSAAM	HUFSA
HOLLY-MARIE	HOSAM	HUFSAH
HOLLY-MAY	HOSANA	HUGAS
HOLLY-ROSE	HOSANNA	HUGH
HOLLYANN	HOSEA	HUGHIE
HOLLYANNE	HOSNA	HUGO
HOLLYE	HOSSAM	HUI
HOLLYMAY	HOSSEIN	HUKAM
HOLY	HOU	HULYA
HOMAIRA	HOUDA	HUMA
HOMAYRA	HOURIA	HUMAAM
HON	HOUSSAM	HUMAH
HONESTY	HOWARD	HUMAID
HONEY	HOWIE	HUMAIMA
HONEY-BELLE	HREHAAN	HUMAIR
HONEY-LEIGH	HRIAN	HUMAIRA
HONEY-LOU	HRIDAAN	HUMAIRAA
HONEY-LOUISE	HRIDAY	HUMAIRAH
HONEY-MAE	HRIDAYA	HUMAM
HONEY-MAI	HRIDHAAN	HUMARA

HUMAYD
HUMAYL
HUMAYRA
HUMAYRAA
HUMAYRAH
HUMAYUN
HUMEIRA
HUMERA
HUMERAH
HUMEYRA
HUMIRA
HUMMA
HUMMERA
HUMNA
HUMNAH
HUMPHREY
HUMPHRY
HUMYRA
HUMZA
HUMZAH
HUNAIN
HUNAYN
HUNG
HUNNI
HUNNIE
HUNNY
HUNOR
HUNTER
HUNTER-JAMES
HUNTER-LEE
HUNTER-RAY
HUNTER-ROSE
HUNTLEY
HURAIN
HURAIRA
HURAIRAH
HURIA
HURIYA
HURIYAH
HURIYYAH
HURLEY
HURR
HURREM
HURSH
HUSAAM
HUSAIN
HUSAINA
HUSAM
HUSAYN
HUSEIN
HUSEYIN
HUSNA
HUSNAA
HUSNAH
HUSNAIN
HUSNAYN
HUSNEIN
HUSNI
HUSSAIN
HUSSAM
HUSSAN
HUSSEIN
HUSSEN
HUSSIEN
HUSSIN
HUSSNA
HUSSNAIN
HUW
HUXLEY
HUY
HUZAIFA
HUZAIFAH
HUZAIR
HUZAYFA
HUZAYFAH
HUZAYL
HUZEFA
HYAB
HYDER
HYDIE
HYLTON
HYRUM
HYUN
HYWEL

I

IACOB
IACOPO
IACOV
IAGO
IAIN
IAN
IAN-JUNIOR
IANA
IANIS
IANNA
IANNIS
IANTHE
IANTO
IARA
IARLA
IASHA
IASMINA
IASON
IASONAS
IBA
IBAAD
IBAD
IBADAH
IBBIE
IBEN
IBIRONKE
IBRAAHEEM
IBRAAHIM
IBRAHEEM
IBRAHEM
IBRAHIIM
IBRAHIM
IBRAHIMA
IBRAR
IBTIHAAL
IBTIHAJ
IBTIHAL
IBTISAAM
IBTISAM
IBTISSAM
IBUKUN
IBUKUNOLUWA
ICE
ICY

IDA
IDA-MAY
IDA-ROSE
IDAL
IDALIA
IDAN
IDARA
IDDO
IDEN
IDIL
IDIRIS
IDMAN
IDNAN
IDO
IDOWU
IDREECE
IDREES
IDRIS
IDRISS
IDRISSA
IEASHA
IEAUN
IEESHA
IEFAN
IEISHA
IESA
IESHA
IESHAA
IESTYN
IEUAN
IEVA
IFAN
IFAT
IFE
IFEANYI
IFEANYICHUKWU
IFECHUKWU
IFECHUKWUDE
IFEDAYO
IFEOLUWA
IFEOLUWAPO
IFEOMA
IFETAYO
IFFAH
IFFAT
IFFATH
IFOR
IFRA

IFRAH
IFRAN
IFRAZ
IFSA
IFSAH
IFTEKAR
IFTEKHAR
IFTIKAR
IFTIKHAR
IFUNANYA
IFUNANYACHUKWU
IFZA
IFZAH
IFZAL
IGA
IGGY
IGLI
IGNACIO
IGNACY
IGNAS
IGNATIUS
IGOR
IHAB
IHFAZ
IHINOSEN
IHSAAN
IHSAN
IHTESHAM
IHTISHAAM
IHTISHAM
IIYLA
IJAAZ
IJAH
IJAZ
IJEOMA
IKE
IKECHI
IKECHUKWU
IKECHUKWUKA
IKEMEFUNA
IKENNA
IKEOLUWA
IKER
IKHLAAS
IKHLAS
IKHRA
IKJOT
IKPONMWOSA

IKRA
IKRAA
IKRAAM
IKRAAN
IKRAH
IKRAM
IKRAN
IKRANUR
ILA
ILA-ROSE
ILAH
ILAI
ILAKKIYA
ILAN
ILANA
ILANAH
ILANI
ILARIA
ILAY
ILAYDA
ILEANA
ILENA
ILENIA
ILERIOLUWA
ILESH
ILHAAM
ILHAAN
ILHAM
ILHAN
ILIA
ILIAN
ILIANA
ILIANNA
ILIAS
ILIE
ILIJA
ILINA
ILINCA
ILIR
ILIRIAN
ILISHA
ILITHYIA
ILIYA
ILIYAN
ILIYANA
ILIYAS
ILIZA
ILJA

ILKAY
ILLAN
ILLANA
ILLEANA
ILLIANA
ILLIANNA
ILLIAS
ILLIYEEN
ILLYA
ILLYANA
ILLYAS
ILMA
ILONA
ILSA
ILSE
ILWAAD
ILWAD
ILYA
ILYAANA
ILYAAS
ILYAN
ILYANA
ILYAS
ILYAZ
ILYES
ILYSSA
IMA
IMAAD
IMAAM
IMAAN
IMAANI
IMAD
IMAGEN
IMAM
IMAMA
IMAMAH
IMAN
IMANA
IMANE
IMANI
IMANI-ROSE
IMANUEL
IMANY
IMARA
IMARAH
IMARI
IMARNI
IMARNIE

IMAYA
IMDAD
IMELDA
IMELIA
IMEN
IMILIA
IMISIOLUWA
IMMACULATE
IMMANUEL
IMMANUELLA
IMMIE
IMMOGEN
IMMY
IMOGEN
IMOGEN-GRACE
IMOGEN-HOPE
IMOGEN-LEIGH
IMOGEN-LOUISE
IMOGEN-MAE
IMOGEN-MAI
IMOGEN-ROSE
IMOGENE
IMOGIN
IMOGINE
IMOJEN
IMRAAN
IMRAN
IMRANA
IMRANUL
IMRE
IMREN
IMTIAZ
IMTITHAL
IMTIYAAZ
IMTIYAZ
INA
INAAM
INAARA
INAAYA
INAAYAH
INABIYAH
INAIYA
INAIYAH
INAM
INAN
INARA
INARAH
INARI

INAS
INAYA
INAYAA
INAYAAH
INAYAH
INAYAT
INCA
INCI
INDAH
INDEA
INDEE
INDEG
INDER
INDERDEEP
INDERJEET
INDERJIT
INDERPAL
INDERPREET
INDERVEER
INDI
INDI-RAE
INDI-ROSE
INDIA
INDIA-LEIGH
INDIA-MAE
INDIA-ROSE
INDIAH
INDIANA
INDIANA-ROSE
INDIANNA
INDICA
INDIE
INDIE-LEIGH
INDIE-MAE
INDIE-MAI
INDIE-MAY
INDIE-RAE
INDIE-ROSE
INDIGO
INDIO
INDIRA
INDIYA
INDIYA-ROSE
INDIYAH
INDRA
INDRAJ
INDRIT
INDY

INDY-ROSE
INDYA
INDYANA
INES
INESA
INESH
INESS
INESSA
INEZ
INGA
INGE
INGO
INGRID
INIGO
INIKA
INIOLUWA
INIYA
INKA
INNA
INNAYA
INNAYAH
INNES
INNIS
INNOCENT
INOLA
INSHA
INSHAAL
INSHIRAH
INSIYA
INSIYAH
INTI
INTISAAR
INTISAR
INZA
IO
IOAN
IOANA
IOANE
IOANNA
IOANNIS
IOLA
IOLANTHE
IOLE
IOLI
IOLO
ION
IONA
IONATAN

IONE
IONEL
IONELA
IONI
IONIE
IONUT
IORI
IORWERTH
IOSIF
IOSUA
IOWA
IPEK
IPTISAM
IQBAAL
IQBAL
IQLAAS
IQLAS
IQRA
IQRAA
IQRAH
IQRAM
IRA
IRAH
IRAJ
IRAM
IRELAND
IREM
IREMIDE
IREMSU
IRENA
IRENE
IRENOSEN
IREOLUWA
IREOLUWATOMIWA
IRETOMIWA
IRFA
IRFAAN
IRFAN
IRHA
IRHAA
IRIE
IRIM
IRINA
IRINI
IRIS
IRIS-LILY
IRIS-ROSE
IRISA

IRMA	ISABELLE	ISHER
IRMAK	ISABELLE-GRACE	ISHFAQ
IROH	ISABELLE-MAE	ISHIKA
IRRAM	ISABELLE-ROSE	ISHITA
IRRUM	ISAC	ISHITHA
IRSA	ISACC	ISHKA
IRSAH	ISADORA	ISHMAEL
IRSHAAD	ISAH	ISHMAIL
IRTAZA	ISAHAK	ISHMAM
IRTIQA	ISAHAQ	ISHMEAL
IRTIZA	ISAIA	ISHMEET
IRUM	ISAIAH	ISHNEET
IRUNDEEP	ISAIAS	ISHPREET
IRVIN	ISAK	ISHRAQ
IRVINE	ISAM	ISHRAT
IRVING	ISAMBARD	ISHRATH
IRWIN	ISAQ	ISHTIAQ
IRYS	ISATA	ISHVEER
IRZA	ISATOU	ISHWAR
IS-HAAQ	ISATU	ISHYA
IS'HAAQ	ISAURA	ISIAH
IS'HAQ	ISAURE	ISIDORA
ISA	ISBAH	ISIDORE
ISAA	ISCHIA	ISIL
ISAAC	ISEABAIL	ISIOMA
ISAAC-JAMES	ISEBELLE	ISIS
ISAAC-JAY	ISEULT	ISKANDER
ISAAC-LEE	ISHA	ISLA
ISAAH	ISHAA	ISLA-
ISAAK	ISHAAC	ISLA-BEAU
ISAAM	ISHAAL	ISLA-BELLE
ISAAQ	ISHAAN	ISLA-FAITH
ISABEAU	ISHAANI	ISLA-GRACE
ISABEL	ISHAAQ	ISLA-JADE
ISABEL-ROSE	ISHAH	ISLA-JANE
ISABELA	ISHAK	ISLA-LILY
ISABELE	ISHAL	ISLA-LOUISE
ISABELL	ISHAN	ISLA-MAE
ISABELLA	ISHANA	ISLA-MAI
ISABELLA-GRACE	ISHANI	ISLA-MARIE
ISABELLA-LOUISE	ISHANVI	ISLA-MAY
ISABELLA-MAE	ISHAQ	ISLA-RAE
ISABELLA-MAI	ISHAQUE	ISLA-RAI
ISABELLA-MAY	ISHAR	ISLA-ROSE
ISABELLA-PAIGE	ISHARA	ISLAH
ISABELLA-RAE	ISHBEL	ISLAM
ISABELLA-ROSE	ISHE	ISLAY
ISABELLAH	ISHEANESU	ISLEY

ISMA	ISSOBELLA	IVY
ISMA'EEL	ISSOBELLE	IVY-ANN
ISMA'IL	ISSRA	IVY-BEAU
ISMAA	ISSY	IVY-BELLE
ISMAA'EEL	ISTVAN	IVY-ELIZABETH
ISMAAEEL	ISYLA	IVY-GRACE
ISMAAEL	ISZAC	IVY-JANE
ISMAE	ITA	IVY-JEAN
ISMAEEL	ITAI	IVY-LEE
ISMAEIL	ITALIA	IVY-LEIGH
ISMAEL	ITAMAR	IVY-LOUISE
ISMAH	ITEOLUWAKISHI	IVY-MAE
ISMAHAN	ITHIEL	IVY-MAI
ISMAIEL	ITHSHAM	IVY-MARIE
ISMAIL	ITOHAN	IVY-MAY
ISMAILA	ITSHAM	IVY-RAE
ISMAT	IUAN	IVY-ROSE
ISMAY	IUDITA	IVY-WILLOW
ISMET	IULIA	IWAN
ISOBEL	IULIAN	IWINOSA
ISOBEL-ROSE	IULIANA	IWO
ISOBELA	IUSTIN	IWONA
ISOBELL	IUSTINA	IXIA
ISOBELLA	IVA	IYA
ISOBELLA-MAE	IVAAN	IYAAD
ISOBELLE	IVAN	IYAAN
ISOLA	IVANA	IYAAS
ISOLDE	IVANAH	IYAAZ
ISRA	IVANDRO	IYAD
ISRAA	IVANKA	IYAH
ISRAAR	IVANNA	IYAN
ISRAEL	IVAR	IYANA
ISRAFIL	IVAYLA	IYANLA
ISRAH	IVAYLO	IYANNA
ISRAR	IVEE	IYANNAH
ISREAL	IVELIN	IYANU
ISSA	IVEN	IYANUOLUWA
ISSABEL	IVER	IYAS
ISSABELL	IVET	IYAZ
ISSABELLA	IVETA	IYESHA
ISSABELLE	IVEY	IYINOLUWA
ISSAC	IVIE	IYLA
ISSAH	IVIE-ROSE	IYLA-GRACE
ISSAK	IVO	IYLA-JANE
ISSAM	IVON	IYLA-MAE
ISSE	IVOR	IYLA-MAI
ISSEY	IVORY	IYLA-MAY
ISSIAH	IVORY-ROSE	IYLA-RAE

IYLA-ROSE
IYLAH
IYLAH-MAE
IYLAH-ROSE
IYMAN
IYOBOSA
IYRA
IYRAH
IYSHA
IYSLA
IYZA
IYZAH
IZA
IZAAC
IZAAK
IZAAN
IZAAZ
IZABEL
IZABELA
IZABELE
IZABELL
IZABELLA
IZABELLA-GRACE
IZABELLA-ROSE
IZABELLE
IZAC
IZACC
IZACK
IZADORA
IZAH
IZAIAH
IZAIYAH
IZAK
IZAN
IZARA
IZARRA
IZAYAH
IZAZUL
IZEL
IZEYAH
IZHAAN
IZHAAR
IZHAN
IZIAH
IZMA
IZNA
IZNAH
IZOBEL
IZOBELLA
IZOBELLE
IZUCHUKWU
IZUMI
IZYAAN
IZYAN
IZZA
IZZABEL
IZZABELL
IZZABELLA
IZZABELLE
IZZAH
IZZAK
IZZAT
IZZET
IZZEY
IZZI
IZZIE
IZZIE-MAE
IZZOBELLA
IZZY
IZZY-MAE
IZZY-MAI
IZZY-MAY

J

J
J-JAY
J-KWON
J.
J'ADORE
J'NAI
J'QUAN
J'ZIAH
JA'NAE
JAABIR
JAAD
JAAFAR
JAAN
JAANA
JAANVI
JAAP
JAAZIAH
JABAR
JABARI
JABBAR
JABE
JABED
JABEEN
JABER
JABEZ
JABIR
JABOU
JABRAAN
JABRAN
JABREEL
JABRIIL
JABRIL
JAC
JACCOB
JACE
JACEE
JACEK
JACELYN
JACEN
JACEY
JACEY-LEIGH
JACEY-MAE
JACHIN
JACI

JACIE
JACINDA
JACINTA
JACINTHA
JACINTO
JACK
JACK-DANIEL
JACK-DEAN
JACK-JAMES
JACK-JUNIOR
JACK-RYAN
JACK-THOMAS
JACKIE
JACKIR
JACKSON
JACKSON-JAMES
JACKSON-LEE
JACKY
JACLYN
JACO
JACOB
JACOB-GEORGE
JACOB-JACK
JACOB-JAMES
JACOB-JAY
JACOB-JOE
JACOB-JOHN
JACOB-JOSEPH
JACOB-LEE
JACOB-SCOTT
JACOBE
JACOBI
JACOBIE
JACOBO
JACOBUS
JACOBY
JACOPO
JACQUE
JACQUELINE
JACQUELYN
JACQUES
JACQUI
JACSON
JACUB
JACY
JAD
JADA
JADA-ROSE

JADAH
JADAINE
JADAN
JADE
JADE-LEE
JADE-LOUISE
JADE-MARIE
JADEAN
JADEEN
JADEN
JADEN-JAMES
JADEN-LEE
JADENE
JADESOLA
JADEY
JADIE
JADIEL
JADINE
JADON
JADORE
JADWIGA
JADYN
JADZIA
JAE
JAEDA
JAEDAN
JAEDEN
JAEDON
JAEDYN
JAEGER
JAEL
JAELA
JAELAN
JAELEN
JAELLE
JAELYN
JAEVON
JAFAR
JAFER
JAFFAR
JAGAN
JAGAT
JAGDEEP
JAGDEV
JAGGER
JAGJEET
JAGJEEVAN
JAGJIT

JAGJOT	JAHMIAH	JAILA
JAGNA	JAHMOY	JAILAN
JAGNOOR	JAHNAE	JAILEN
JAGO	JAHNAI	JAILON
JAGODA	JAHNAVI	JAIMA
JAGPAL	JAHNAY	JAIMAL
JAGPREET	JAHNAYAH	JAIMAN
JAGRAJ	JAHNI	JAIME
JAGROOP	JAHNIAH	JAIME-LEA
JAGTAR	JAHNVI	JAIME-LEE
JAGVEER	JAHNYAH	JAIME-LEIGH
JAGVIR	JAHREL	JAIME-LOUISE
JAHAAN	JAHRELL	JAIMEE
JAHAN	JAHROME	JAIMEE-LEE
JAHANARA	JAHSIAH	JAIMEE-LEIGH
JAHANGIR	JAHVANI	JAIMES
JAHANZAIB	JAHVARI	JAIMESON
JAHANZEB	JAHVARN	JAIMEY
JAHARI	JAHVARNI	JAIMI
JAHAZIEL	JAHVEL	JAIMIE
JAHDEL	JAHVON	JAIMIE-LEIGH
JAHDELL	JAHVONTE	JAIMIN
JAHED	JAHZARA	JAIMINI
JAHEDUR	JAHZARAH	JAINA
JAHEEM	JAHZIAH	JAINABA
JAHEIM	JAI	JAINAM
JAHI	JAI-JAI	JAINEEL
JAHID	JAIA	JAINI
JAHIDA	JAICE	JAINIL
JAHIDUL	JAICEE	JAINISH
JAHIDUR	JAICOB	JAIPAL
JAHIEM	JAID	JAIPREET
JAHIME	JAIDA	JAIRAJ
JAHIN	JAIDAH	JAIRUS
JAHIR	JAIDAN	JAISAL
JAHKAI	JAIDAN-LEE	JAISEN
JAHKYE	JAIDE	JAISEY
JAHLEEL	JAIDEEP	JAISHA
JAHMAI	JAIDEN	JAISHNA
JAHMAINE	JAIDEN-JAMES	JAISON
JAHMAL	JAIDEN-LEE	JAITON
JAHMALI	JAIDEV	JAIVAL
JAHMANI	JAIDIE	JAIVAN
JAHMAR	JAIDON	JAIVEER
JAHMARI	JAIDYN	JAIVEN
JAHMARNI	JAIGO	JAIVIN
JAHMEL	JAIK	JAIVIR
JAHMENE	JAIKE	JAIVON

JAIVYN	JAMARI	JAMIL
JAIYA	JAMARIO	JAMILA
JAIYAH	JAMARL	JAMILAH
JAIYAN	JAMARLEY	JAMILIA
JAIYANA	JAMAUL	JAMILLA
JAIYDEN	JAMAYNE	JAMIMA
JAIYEOLA	JAMEE	JAMIN
JAK	JAMEEL	JAMINA
JAKE	JAMEELA	JAMISON
JAKE-JAMES	JAMEELAH	JAMIUL
JAKE-JUNIOR	JAMEIL	JAMMAL
JAKE-LEE	JAMEL	JAMOY
JAKEY	JAMELA	JAN
JAKIA	JAMELAH	JAN-MICHAEL
JAKIR	JAMELIA	JANA
JAKK	JAMELL	JANADE
JAKKE	JAMES	JANAE
JAKOB	JAMES-ANTHONY	JANAH
JAKOBI	JAMES-DEAN	JANAI
JAKOBUS	JAMES-JOHN	JANAID
JAKOBY	JAMES-JUNIOR	JANAK
JAKSON	JAMES-LEE	JANAKI
JAKUB	JAMES-THOMAS	JANAN
JALAAL	JAMESDEAN	JANANI
JALAL	JAMESON	JANAT
JALE	JAMEY	JANAV
JALEEL	JAMI	JANAVI
JALEES	JAMIA	JANAY
JALEN	JAMIAH	JANAYA
JALIA	JAMIE	JANAYAH
JALIL	JAMIE-	JANE
JALILA	JAMIE-ANN	JANEETA
JALILAH	JAMIE-DEAN	JANEK
JALIYAH	JAMIE-JOHN	JANEL
JAMA	JAMIE-JUNIOR	JANELL
JAMAAL	JAMIE-LEA	JANELLA
JAMAHL	JAMIE-LEE	JANELLE
JAMAI	JAMIE-LEI	JANESSA
JAMAICA	JAMIE-LEIGH	JANET
JAMAIMA	JAMIE-LOUISE	JANETTE
JAMAIN	JAMIE-SCOTT	JANEY
JAMAINE	JAMIEE	JANGEER
JAMAL	JAMIEL	JANI
JAMALI	JAMIELEA	JANIA
JAMALL	JAMIELEE	JANIAH
JAMALLE	JAMIELEIGH	JANICE
JAMANI	JAMIESON	JANIE
JAMAR	JAMIKA	JANIKA

JANINA
JANINE
JANIS
JANISHA
JANITA
JANIYA
JANIYAH
JANKA
JANKI
JANNA
JANNAH
JANNAI
JANNAT
JANNATH
JANNATPREET
JANNATUL
JANNATUN
JANNEKE
JANNET
JANNI
JANOS
JANOSHAN
JANSEN
JANSI
JANSON
JANUJAN
JANUSH
JANUSHA
JANUSHAN
JANUSZ
JANVI
JANYA
JANZEN
JAPHET
JAPHETH
JAPJI
JAPJIT
JAPLEEN
JAPMAN
JAPNEET
JAPNOOR
JAPVEER
JAQ
JAQUAN
JAQUE
JAQUELINE
JAQUES
JARA

JARAD
JARDEL
JARDELL
JARED
JARED-JAMES
JAREK
JAREL
JARELL
JAREN
JARET
JARETH
JARI
JARIN
JARIYAH
JARLATH
JARNAIL
JARNO
JAROD
JAROM
JAROME
JARON
JAROSLAV
JAROSLAVA
JAROSLAW
JARRAD
JARRED
JARRELL
JARREN
JARRET
JARRETT
JARROD
JARRON
JARRYD
JARVIS
JARYD
JAS
JASBIR
JASDEEP
JASDEV
JASE
JASEENA
JASEMIN
JASEY
JASGUN
JASH
JASHAN
JASHANDEEP
JASHANPREET

JASIA
JASIAH
JASIEL
JASIKA
JASIM
JASIR
JASJEET
JASJOT
JASKARAN
JASKARN
JASKEERAT
JASKIRAN
JASKIRAT
JASKIRIT
JASLEEN
JASLENE
JASLYN
JASMAN
JASMEEN
JASMEET
JASMIA
JASMIN
JASMINA
JASMINDER
JASMINE
JASMINE-JADE
JASMINE-LEIGH
JASMINE-ROSE
JASMINKA
JASMIRA
JASMYN
JASMYNE
JASNEET
JASNOOR
JASON
JASON-JAMES
JASON-JUNIOR
JASON-LEE
JASPA
JASPAL
JASPAR
JASPER
JASPREET
JASPRIT
JASPRIYA
JASRAH
JASRAJ
JASREEN

JASREET	JAVON	JAYCEE-LEE
JASROOP	JAVONE	JAYCEE-LEIGH
JASSER	JAVONTAE	JAYCEE-MAE
JASSICA	JAVONTE	JAYCEN
JASSIM	JAWAAD	JAYCEON
JASTIN	JAWAD	JAYCEY
JASVEEN	JAWAHER	JAYCI
JASVEER	JAWAHIR	JAYCIE
JASVINDER	JAWAIRIA	JAYCIE-LEIGH
JASVIR	JAWAIRIYA	JAYCOB
JASWANT	JAWARIA	JAYCUB
JASWINDER	JAWDAN	JAYD
JATHUSAN	JAWERIA	JAYDA
JATHUSHA	JAWERIYA	JAYDAH
JATHUSHAN	JAWHARA	JAYDAN
JATIN	JAWWAD	JAYDAN-LEE
JATINDER	JAX	JAYDE
JAVAD	JAXEN	JAYDEAN
JAVAE	JAXON	JAYDEE
JAVAID	JAXON-JAMES	JAYDEEN
JAVAIRIA	JAXON-JOHN	JAYDEEP
JAVAN	JAXON-LEE	JAYDEN
JAVANI	JAXSON	JAYDEN-CRUZ
JAVANIE	JAXSON-JAMES	JAYDEN-JAMES
JAVANNI	JAXSON-JAY	JAYDEN-JAY
JAVANTE	JAXSON-LEE	JAYDEN-JOHN
JAVARI	JAXTON	JAYDEN-LEE
JAVARIA	JAXX	JAYDEN-LEIGH
JAVARN	JAXXON	JAYDEN-LEWIS
JAVARNE	JAY	JAYDEN-PAUL
JAVARNI	JAY-	JAYDENE
JAVAUGHN	JAY-D	JAYDEV
JAVAUN	JAY-DEE	JAYDINE
JAVED	JAY-J	JAYDN
JAVEL	JAY-JAMES	JAYDON
JAVELL	JAY-JAY	JAYDYN
JAVEN	JAY-JUNIOR	JAYE
JAVENE	JAY-LEE	JAYED
JAVERIA	JAYA	JAYEN
JAVERIAH	JAYAH	JAYESH
JAVERIYA	JAYAN	JAYGO
JAVI	JAYANA	JAYIN
JAVID	JAYANI	JAYJAY
JAVIER	JAYANNA	JAYK
JAVIN	JAYANT	JAYKE
JAVINA	JAYANTH	JAYKOB
JAVINE	JAYCE	JAYKUB
JAVION	JAYCEE	JAYLA

JAYLA-MAI
JAYLAH
JAYLAN
JAYLEA
JAYLEE
JAYLEEN
JAYLEIGH
JAYLEN
JAYLIN
JAYLON
JAYME
JAYME-LEE
JAYME-LEIGH
JAYMEE
JAYMEE-LEIGH
JAYMES
JAYMI
JAYMI-LEIGH
JAYMIE
JAYMIE-LEE
JAYMIE-LEIGH
JAYMIE-LOUISE
JAYMIN
JAYMZ
JAYNA
JAYNE
JAYNI
JAYNIE
JAYON
JAYQUAN
JAYRAJ
JAYRON
JAYSE
JAYSEN
JAYSON
JAYVEER
JAYVEN
JAYVION
JAYVIR
JAYVON
JAZ
JAZAIAH
JAZARA
JAZIAH
JAZIB
JAZIBA
JAZIEL
JAZLEEN

JAZLYN
JAZMIN
JAZMINE
JAZMYN
JAZMYNE
JAZZ
JAZZLYN
JAZZMIN
JAZZMINE
JAZZMYN
JEAN
JEAN-
JEAN-BAPTISTE
JEAN-CLAUDE
JEAN-JACQUES
JEAN-LOUIS
JEAN-LUC
JEAN-PAUL
JEAN-PIERRE
JEANA
JEANELLE
JEANETTE
JEANIE
JEANINE
JEANNA
JEANNE
JEANNETTE
JEANNIE
JEBA
JED
JEDAIAH
JEDD
JEDEDIAH
JEDIAH
JEDIDAH
JEDIDIAH
JEDRZEJ
JEEL
JEENA
JEET
JEEVA
JEEVAN
JEEVANSH
JEEVAT
JEEVEN
JEEVIKA
JEEVUN
JEEYA

JEFF
JEFFERSON
JEFFERY
JEFFREY
JEGORS
JEHAD
JEHAN
JEHIEL
JEHOVANI
JEHU
JEKABS
JELANI
JELENA
JELIZAVETA
JEM
JEMA
JEMAINE
JEMAL
JEMEL
JEMEMAH
JEMI
JEMIAH
JEMILA
JEMIMA
JEMIMAH
JEMINA
JEMINI
JEMMA
JEMMA-LOUISE
JEMMIMA
JEMUEL
JEN
JENA
JENADE
JENAE
JENAI
JENAN
JENARA
JENAY
JENAYA
JENAYAH
JENEBA
JENELL
JENELLE
JENESSA
JENEVIEVE
JENI
JENIA

JENICA
JENICE
JENIFER
JENIKA
JENIL
JENIN
JENINE
JENISH
JENISHA
JENITA
JENKIN
JENNA
JENNA-LEIGH
JENNA-LOUISE
JENNAH
JENNAYA
JENNER
JENNI
JENNICA
JENNIE
JENNIFER
JENNIFER-ROSE
JENNIKA
JENNY
JENS
JENSEN
JENSEN-JAMES
JENSON
JENSON-JAMES
JENSON-JAY
JENSON-JOHN
JENSON-JOSEPH
JENSON-LEE
JEORGE
JEORGIA
JEORGIE
JERAHMEEL
JERALD
JERAMIAH
JERED
JERELL
JEREMI
JEREMIAH
JEREMIASZ
JEREMIE
JEREMIH
JEREMY
JERI

JERIAH
JERICA
JERICHO
JERIEL
JERIMIAH
JERMAIN
JERMAINE
JERMAYNE
JERMIAH
JEROEN
JEROME
JERON
JERONE
JERRARD
JERREL
JERRELL
JERRY
JERSEY
JERSEY-LOU
JERSEY-RAE
JERSI
JERSIE
JERUSALEM
JERUSHA
JERZIE
JERZY
JESAIAH
JESAL
JESAMINE
JESCA
JESHAN
JESHUA
JESHURUN
JESIAH
JESICA
JESIKA
JESKA
JESLIN
JESLYN
JESMIN
JESPER
JESS
JESSA
JESSALYN
JESSAME
JESSAMIE
JESSAMINE
JESSAMY

JESSAMYN
JESSE
JESSE-JAMES
JESSE-JOE
JESSE-LEE
JESSECA
JESSENIA
JESSEY
JESSI
JESSIAH
JESSICA
JESSICA-
JESSICA-ANNE
JESSICA-GRACE
JESSICA-JADE
JESSICA-JANE
JESSICA-JAY
JESSICA-JAYNE
JESSICA-LEA
JESSICA-LEE
JESSICA-LEIGH
JESSICA-LILLY
JESSICA-LILY
JESSICA-LOUISE
JESSICA-MAE
JESSICA-MAI
JESSICA-MARIE
JESSICA-MAY
JESSICA-PAIGE
JESSICA-ROSE
JESSICA-TAYLOR
JESSICCA
JESSIE
JESSIE-ANNE
JESSIE-JAMES
JESSIE-LEE
JESSIE-LEIGH
JESSIE-MAE
JESSIE-MAI
JESSIE-MAY
JESSIE-RAE
JESSIE-ROSE
JESSIKA
JESSIKAH
JESSY
JESSYCA
JESSYE
JESTON

JESUS
JESUTOFUNMI
JESWIN
JET
JETA
JETHRO
JETMIR
JETON
JETSON
JETT
JETTA
JEVAN
JEVAUGHN
JEVEN
JEVIN
JEVON
JEVONTE
JEWEL
JEWELL
JEYA
JEYDA
JEYHAN
JEYLAN
JEZ
JEZIAH
JEZREEL
JEZZ
JHANAE
JHANE
JHANGIR
JHANVI
JHENE
JHNELLE
JHON
JI
JIA
JIAH
JIAHAO
JIAHUI
JIAN
JIANA
JIANG
JIANNA
JIAQI
JIAWEI
JIAYI
JIAYUE
JIBRAAN
JIBRAEEL
JIBRAEL
JIBRAIL
JIBRAN
JIBREEL
JIBRIEL
JIBRIIL
JIBRIL
JIDENNA
JIE
JIGAR
JIHAAN
JIHAD
JIHAN
JILL
JILLIAN
JILLY
JIM
JIMENA
JIMI
JIMMI
JIMMIE
JIMMY
JIMMY-DEAN
JIMMY-JAMES
JIMMY-JOE
JIMMY-LEE
JIMMY-RAY
JIN
JINA
JINAL
JINAN
JINAY
JINESH
JING
JINNY
JIORDAN
JIRAIYA
JIREH
JIRI
JIRO
JISHA
JISHNU
JITEN
JITESH
JIVAN
JIVIN
JIVRAJ
JIYA
JIYAAD
JIYAAN
JIYAN
JIYANA
JJ
JO
JO-ANN
JO-ANNA
JO-ANNE
JO-LEIGH
JOAB
JOACHIM
JOAH
JOAKIM
JOAL
JOAN
JOANA
JOANI
JOANIE
JOANN
JOANNA
JOANNAH
JOANNE
JOAO
JOAQUIM
JOAQUIN
JOASH
JOB
JOBAN
JOBE
JOBEN
JOBEY
JOBI
JOBIE
JOBY
JOCASTA
JOCCOAA
JOCELIN
JOCELYN
JOCELYNE
JOCHEBED
JOCIE
JOCK
JODEE
JODEN
JODENE
JODH

JODHI
JODHVEER
JODI
JODI-LEIGH
JODIE
JODIE-ANN
JODIE-LEE
JODIE-LEIGH
JODIE-MAE
JODIE-MAY
JODINE
JODY
JOE
JOE-LEWIS
JOEB
JOEL
JOELI
JOELIE
JOELL
JOELLA
JOELLE
JOELY
JOEN
JOESEPH
JOESPH
JOEY
JOEY-JAMES
JOEY-JAY
JOEY-LEE
JOHAAN
JOHAN
JOHANA
JOHANAN
JOHANN
JOHANNA
JOHANNAH
JOHANNES
JOHARA
JOHB
JOHIRUL
JOHN
JOHN-
JOHN-BOY
JOHN-FRANCIS
JOHN-HENRY
JOHN-JACK
JOHN-JAMES
JOHN-JOE

JOHN-JOSEPH
JOHN-JUNIOR
JOHN-LUKE
JOHN-MICHAEL
JOHN-PATRICK
JOHN-PAUL
JOHN-RILEY
JOHN-ROBERT
JOHN-TERRY
JOHN-THOMAS
JOHN-WILLIAM
JOHNATHAN
JOHNATHON
JOHNBOY
JOHNIE
JOHNJAMES
JOHNJOE
JOHNLEE
JOHNNIE
JOHNNY
JOHNNY-LEE
JOHNOTHAN
JOHNPAUL
JOHNSON
JOHNWILLIAM
JOHNY
JOHURA
JOIA
JOIE
JOJO
JOKUBAS
JOLAN
JOLANDA
JOLANTA
JOLE
JOLEE
JOLEEN
JOLEIGH
JOLENE
JOLEON
JOLEY
JOLIE
JOLIN
JOLON
JOLYON
JOMANA
JON
JON-JAMES

JON-LUC
JON-LUKE
JON-PAUL
JONA
JONAH
JONAH-JAMES
JONAID
JONAN
JONAS
JONASZ
JONATAN
JONATHAN
JONATHAN-JAMES
JONATHON
JONEL
JONELLE
JONES
JONI
JONIE
JONJO
JONJOE
JONNIE
JONNY
JONO
JONOTHAN
JONPAUL
JONSON
JONTE
JONTI
JONTY
JOO
JOOD
JOOLS
JOORY
JOOST
JORA
JORAM
JORAWAR
JORDACHE
JORDAINE
JORDAN
JORDAN-JAMES
JORDAN-JUNIOR
JORDAN-LEE
JORDAN-LEIGH
JORDAN-REECE
JORDANA
JORDANE

JORDANLEE	JOSE	JOSS
JORDANN	JOSEF	JOSSELIN
JORDANNA	JOSEFF	JOSSELYN
JORDANNE	JOSEFIN	JOSSLYN
JORDELL	JOSEFINA	JOSUA
JORDELLE	JOSEFINE	JOSUAH
JORDEN	JOSELYN	JOSUE
JORDI	JOSEPH	JOSUHA
JORDIE	JOSEPH-JACK	JOTHAM
JORDIN	JOSEPH-JAMES	JOUD
JORDINA	JOSEPH-JOHN	JOUDY
JORDON	JOSEPH-JUNIOR	JOULES
JORDON-LEE	JOSEPH-LEE	JOUMANA
JORDY	JOSEPHA	JOURDAIN
JORDYN	JOSEPHINA	JOURDAN
JORE	JOSEPHINE	JOURI
JOREL	JOSETTE	JOURNEY
JORELL	JOSEY	JOURY
JORGA	JOSH	JOVAIRIA
JORGE	JOSHAN	JOVAN
JORGEN	JOSHIKA	JOVANA
JORGI	JOSHIM	JOVANI
JORGIA	JOSHKUN	JOVANNI
JORGIANA	JOSHPAL	JOVANNY
JORGIE	JOSHUA	JOVAWN
JORGIE-LEA	JOSHUA-	JOVEN
JORGIE-LEIGH	JOSHUA-DAVID	JOVI
JORGIE-MAE	JOSHUA-JAMES	JOVIAN
JORGIE-MAI	JOSHUA-JAY	JOVIE
JORGIE-MAY	JOSHUA-JOHN	JOVIN
JORGIE-RAE	JOSHUA-JUNIOR	JOVITA
JORGIE-ROSE	JOSHUA-LEE	JOVUN
JORGINA	JOSHUA-LEWIS	JOWAN
JORI	JOSHUAH	JOWEN
JORIS	JOSHVEER	JOWITA
JORJ	JOSHWA	JOY
JORJA	JOSI	JOYA
JORJA-LEIGH	JOSIA	JOYCE
JORJA-MAE	JOSIAH	JOYCELYN
JORJA-MAY	JOSIANE	JOYNUL
JORJA-ROSE	JOSIAS	JOZEF
JORJI	JOSIE	JOZEFINA
JORJIA	JOSIE-LEA	JOZEPH
JORJIE	JOSIE-LEIGH	JOZIAH
JORY	JOSIE-MAE	JOZSEF
JOS	JOSIE-MARIE	JU
JOSCELINE	JOSIE-MAY	JUAN
JOSCELYN	JOSLYN	JUANA

JUANITA
JUANNA
JUBAIR
JUBAL
JUBAYDAH
JUBAYER
JUBEDA
JUBEL
JUBER
JUBILEE
JUBRIL
JUD
JUDAH
JUDD
JUDE
JUDGE
JUDI
JUDIE
JUDITH
JUDY
JUDYTA
JUEL
JUELS
JUELZ
JUGAAD
JUGRAJ
JUHAINA
JUHEL
JUHENA
JUHI
JUI
JUJHAR
JUKE
JULEKHA
JULEN
JULES
JULIA
JULIAN
JULIANA
JULIANE
JULIANNA
JULIANNE
JULIANO
JULIDE
JULIE
JULIE-ANN
JULIE-ANNE
JULIEANN

JULIEANNE
JULIEN
JULIENNE
JULIET
JULIETA
JULIETTA
JULIETTE
JULIJA
JULIO
JULITA
JULIUS
JULIUSZ
JULLIAN
JUMA
JUMAIMA
JUMAIMAH
JUMAINA
JUMAINAH
JUMAN
JUMANA
JUMANAH
JUMARA
JUMAYMAH
JUMEIRAH
JUN
JUNA
JUNAD
JUNAED
JUNAID
JUNAINA
JUNAINAH
JUNAYD
JUNAYNAH
JUNE
JUNED
JUNG
JUNHAO
JUNIA
JUNIOR
JUNIOR-JAMES
JUNIOR-JAY
JUNIPER
JUNKAI
JUNO
JUPITER
JURAJ
JURAN
JURELL

JURGEN
JURI
JUSTAS
JUSTE
JUSTICE
JUSTIN
JUSTIN-JAMES
JUSTIN-LEE
JUSTINA
JUSTINAS
JUSTINE
JUSTIS
JUSTUS
JUSTYN
JUSTYNA
JUSUF
JUVAN
JUVERIA
JUVRAJ
JUWAIRIA
JUWAIRIAH
JUWAIRIYA
JUWAIRIYAH
JUWAIRIYYAH
JUWAIRYAH
JUWAIRYYAH
JUWARIAH
JUWARIYA
JUWARIYAH
JUWAYRIA
JUWAYRIAH
JUWAYRIYA
JUWAYRIYAH
JUWAYRIYYA
JUWAYRIYYAH
JUWERIA
JUWERIYA
JUWEYRIYA
JWANA
JYE
JYOTI
JYOTSNA

K

K
K-CI
K-JAY
KA
KAAJAL
KAAMIL
KAAMILAH
KAAN
KAASHIF
KAASHVI
KAAVIYA
KAAVYA
KAAYA
KAAYAN
KABE
KABEER
KABEL
KABILAN
KABIR
KABIRA
KABISHA
KABISHAN
KABISHAYAN
KACE
KACEE
KACEY
KACEY-
KACEY-ANN
KACEY-JADE
KACEY-JANE
KACEY-JO
KACEY-LEA
KACEY-LEE
KACEY-LEIGH
KACEY-LOUISE
KACEY-MAE
KACEY-MAI
KACEY-MARIE
KACEY-MAY
KACEYLEIGH
KACI
KACI-JANE
KACI-JO
KACI-LEA
KACI-LEE
KACI-LEI
KACI-LEIGH
KACI-LOUISE
KACI-MAE
KACI-MAI
KACI-MARIE
KACI-MAY
KACIA
KACIE
KACIE-ANN
KACIE-JO
KACIE-LEA
KACIE-LEE
KACIE-LEIGH
KACIE-LOUISE
KACIE-MAE
KACIE-MAI
KACIE-MARIE
KACIE-MAY
KACIE-ROSE
KACPER
KACY
KACY-LEIGH
KACY-MAY
KADAN
KADDY
KADE
KADEE
KADEEM
KADEER
KADEJA
KADELL
KADEN
KADEN-JAMES
KADENCE
KADESHA
KADEY
KADEY-LEIGH
KADI
KADI-LEIGH
KADIAN
KADIATOU
KADIATU
KADIDIA
KADIDJA
KADIE
KADIE-LEA
KADIE-LEE
KADIE-LEI
KADIE-LEIGH
KADIE-MAE
KADIE-MAY
KADIELEIGH
KADIJA
KADIJAH
KADIJAT
KADIJATU
KADIN
KADIR
KADISHA
KADIZA
KADMIEL
KADON
KADRA
KADY
KADY-LEA
KADY-LEIGH
KADYN
KAE
KAEDAN
KAEDE
KAEDEN
KAEDON
KAEDYN
KAEL
KAELA
KAELAH
KAELAM
KAELAN
KAELEB
KAELEM
KAELEN
KAELI
KAELIE
KAELIN
KAELON
KAELUM
KAELUN
KAELYN
KAEMON
KAENAN
KAESHA
KAESON
KAETLYN
KAEYA

KAFIA
KAGAN
KAGE
KAH
KAHAN
KAHEESHA
KAHIL
KAHINA
KAHLAN
KAHLEN
KAHLIA
KAHLIL
KAI
KAI-JAMES
KAI-MCKENZIE
KAI-REECE
KAIA
KAIAH
KAIAN
KAIANNA
KAICEE
KAICEY
KAID
KAIDA
KAIDAN
KAIDE
KAIDEE
KAIDEN
KAIDEN-JAMES
KAIDEN-JAY
KAIDEN-LEE
KAIDEN-SCOTT
KAIDENCE
KAIDI
KAIDIE
KAIDON
KAIDY
KAIDYN
KAIE
KAIEN
KAIESHA
KAIF
KAIHAN
KAII
KAIJA
KAIL
KAILA
KAILAH

KAILAM
KAILAN
KAILANI
KAILAS
KAILASH
KAILEB
KAILEE
KAILEIGH
KAILEM
KAILEN
KAILEY
KAILIB
KAILIN
KAILLUM
KAILO
KAILON
KAILUB
KAILUM
KAILUN
KAILYN
KAIM
KAIMANA
KAIMEN
KAIN
KAINA
KAINAAT
KAINAN
KAINAT
KAINE
KAINEN
KAIO
KAIOH
KAION
KAIRA
KAIRAH
KAIRAN
KAIRAV
KAIREECE
KAIRELL
KAIREN
KAIRESE
KAIRI
KAIRO
KAIRON
KAIROS
KAIRYN
KAIS
KAISAAN

KAISAN
KAISAR
KAISEN
KAISER
KAISEY
KAISHA
KAISIE
KAISON
KAITIE
KAITLAN
KAITLAND
KAITLEN
KAITLIN
KAITLIN-LOUISE
KAITLIN-ROSE
KAITLYN
KAITLYN-MARIE
KAITLYN-ROSE
KAITLYNE
KAITLYNN
KAITLYNNE
KAITO
KAIUS
KAIYA
KAIYAAN
KAIYAH
KAIYAN
KAIYEN
KAIYON
KAIZ
KAIZAR
KAIZEN
KAIZER
KAJ
KAJA
KAJAL
KAJAN
KAJETAN
KAJOL
KAJUS
KAL
KAL-EL
KALA
KALAM
KALAN
KALANI
KALAYA
KALDEN

KALE	KALLIE	KAMARL
KALEA	KALLIOPI	KAMARLEY
KALEAH	KALLIS	KAMARLI
KALEB	KALLISTA	KAMARNI
KALEBH	KALLON	KAMAU
KALEE	KALLUM	KAMAYA
KALEEL	KALLY	KAMDEN
KALEEM	KALMAN	KAMEA
KALEESI	KALO	KAMEEL
KALEIGH	KALON	KAMEELA
KALEISHA	KALONICE	KAMEL
KALEL	KALONJI	KAMELIA
KALEM	KALOYAN	KAMEN
KALEN	KALP	KAMERAN
KALESHA	KALSOOM	KAMERON
KALEY	KALSUM	KAMESHA
KALI	KALTHUM	KAMI
KALIA	KALTRINA	KAMIAH
KALIAH	KALU	KAMIL
KALIB	KALUB	KAMILA
KALICE	KALUM	KAMILAH
KALICIA	KALUP	KAMILE
KALID	KALVIN	KAMILIA
KALIE	KALVYN	KAMILIS
KALIF	KALYA	KAMILLA
KALIFA	KALYAN	KAMILYA
KALIL	KALYANI	KAMIRA
KALILA	KALYN	KAMIRAH
KALIM	KAM	KAMISHA
KALIN	KAM'RON	KAMIYA
KALINA	KAMA	KAMIYAH
KALISA	KAMAAL	KAMRAAN
KALISE	KAMAHL	KAMRAN
KALISHA	KAMAI	KAMREN
KALISI	KAMAL	KAMRON
KALISSA	KAMALA	KAMRUL
KALISTA	KAMALDEEP	KAMRUN
KALIYAH	KAMALI	KAMRYN
KALKIDAN	KAMALJEET	KAMSI
KALLAI	KAMALJIT	KAMSIYOCHI
KALLAM	KAMALPREET	KAMSIYOCHUKWU
KALLAN	KAMANI	KAMURAN
KALLE	KAMAR	KAMYA
KALLEL	KAMARA	KAMYAR
KALLEM	KAMARAN	KANA
KALLEN	KAMARI	KANAAN
KALLI	KAMARIA	KANAKO
KALLIA	KAMARION	KANAN

KANAV
KANDI
KANDICE
KANE
KANEEZ
KANG
KANHAIYA
KANI
KANIHA
KANIKA
KANISH
KANISHA
KANISHK
KANISHKA
KANITA
KANIZ
KANNA
KANNAN
KANO
KANON
KANWAL
KANWAR
KANY
KANYA
KANYE
KANYINSOLA
KANZA
KANZAH
KAORI
KAPIL
KAPILAN
KAPRICE
KAR
KARA
KARA-LEIGH
KARA-LOUISE
KARA-ROSE
KARAGH
KARAH
KARALEE
KARAM
KARAMBA
KARAMDEEP
KARAMJEET
KARAMJIT
KARAMVEER
KARAMVIR
KARAN
KARANBIR
KARANDEEP
KARANJEET
KARANJIT
KARANJOT
KARANVEER
KARANVIR
KARAS
KARDEL
KARDELEN
KARDELL
KARDIN
KARDO
KAREEM
KAREEMA
KAREEMAH
KAREEN
KAREENA
KAREL
KARELL
KAREM
KAREN
KARENA
KARENJIT
KARENZA
KARHA
KARHYS
KARI
KARIKALAN
KARILE
KARIM
KARIMA
KARIMAH
KARIN
KARINA
KARINE
KARIS
KARISH
KARISHA
KARISHMA
KARISMA
KARISS
KARISSA
KARL
KARLA
KARLEE
KARLEEN
KARLEIGH
KARLENE
KARLEY
KARLI
KARLIE
KARLINA
KARLIS
KARLO
KARLOS
KARLOTTA
KARLTON
KARLY
KARMA
KARMAN
KARMANI
KARMANJOT
KARMEL
KARMELLA
KARMEN
KARN
KARNA
KARNAN
KARNEL
KARNELL
KARNYE
KARO
KAROL
KAROLINA
KAROLINE
KAROLIS
KARRA
KARRAN
KARRERA
KARRI
KARRIE
KARRIGAN
KARRINA
KARRIS
KARSEN
KARSON
KARSTEN
KARTA
KARTAR
KARTEL
KARTER
KARTHI
KARTHIK
KARTHIKA
KARTHIKEYA

KARTIK
KARUM
KARUN
KARYN
KARYS
KASAM
KASANDRA
KASE
KASEEM
KASEN
KASEY
KASEY-LEE
KASEY-LEIGH
KASEY-MAE
KASEY-MAY
KASH
KASHA
KASHAAN
KASHAF
KASHAI
KASHAN
KASHANE
KASHAUN
KASHEF
KASHI
KASHIF
KASHIFA
KASHISH
KASHMALA
KASHMIR
KASHVI
KASHVIN
KASI
KASIA
KASIAH
KASIAN
KASIB
KASIE
KASIM
KASJAN
KASON
KASPAR
KASPARAS
KASPER
KASPIAN
KASRA
KASS
KASSA

KASSAM
KASSANDRA
KASSEM
KASSEY
KASSI
KASSIA
KASSIAH
KASSIDY
KASSIE
KASSIM
KASSIUS
KASTHURI
KASTURI
KASUMI
KATA
KATALEA
KATALEJA
KATALEYA
KATALIA
KATALIN
KATALINA
KATAN
KATANA
KATARINA
KATARZYNA
KATAYA
KATE
KATE-LYN
KATE-LYNN
KATEE
KATELAN
KATELAND
KATELEN
KATELIN
KATELYN
KATELYN-ROSE
KATELYND
KATELYNE
KATELYNN
KATELYNNE
KATERINA
KATERYNA
KATEY
KATHAN
KATHARINA
KATHARINE
KATHARYN
KATHERINA

KATHERINE
KATHERYN
KATHERYNE
KATHIR
KATHLEEN
KATHLEEN-MARIE
KATHLYN
KATHRIN
KATHRINA
KATHRINE
KATHRYN
KATHRYNE
KATHY
KATI
KATIA
KATIE
KATIE-
KATIE-ANN
KATIE-ANNE
KATIE-GRACE
KATIE-JANE
KATIE-JAYNE
KATIE-JO
KATIE-LEA
KATIE-LEE
KATIE-LEIGH
KATIE-LOU
KATIE-LOUISE
KATIE-MAE
KATIE-MAI
KATIE-MARIE
KATIE-MAY
KATIE-ROSE
KATIEANN
KATIEANNE
KATIELEIGH
KATIELOUISE
KATINKA
KATISHA
KATJA
KATLAN
KATLIN
KATLYN
KATLYNN
KATNISS
KATREENA
KATRESE
KATRIANA

KATRIEL	KAVLEEN	KAYDIE
KATRIN	KAVNEET	KAYDIE-LEIGH
KATRINA	KAVNOOR	KAYDIN
KATRINE	KAVYA	KAYDN
KATRIONA	KAWSAR	KAYDON
KATRYN	KAWTAR	KAYDON-JAY
KATRYNA	KAWTHAR	KAYDY
KATY	KAWTHER	KAYE
KATY-JAYNE	KAY	KAYEL
KATY-LEE	KAY-LEIGH	KAYEN
KATY-LEIGH	KAYA	KAYENAT
KATY-LOUISE	KAYAAN	KAYETAN
KATY-MAY	KAYAH	KAYHAN
KATYA	KAYAHAN	KAYIN
KAUA	KAYAL	KAYJAH
KAUAN	KAYAN	KAYLA
KAUSAR	KAYANA	KAYLA-JAI
KAUSER	KAYANN	KAYLA-LEIGH
KAUSHAL	KAYANNA	KAYLA-LOUISE
KAUSHIK	KAYANNE	KAYLA-MAE
KAUTHAR	KAYCE	KAYLA-MAI
KAVALI	KAYCEE	KAYLA-MARIE
KAVALLI	KAYCEE-LEIGH	KAYLA-MAY
KAVAN	KAYCEE-MAI	KAYLA-ROSE
KAVANA	KAYCEE-MAY	KAYLAB
KAVANAGH	KAYCEY	KAYLAH
KAVARI	KAYCI	KAYLAM
KAVARN	KAYCIE	KAYLAN
KAVARNI	KAYCIE-LEIGH	KAYLANI
KAVEEN	KAYCIE-MARIE	KAYLE
KAVEER	KAYD	KAYLEA
KAVEETA	KAYDA	KAYLEB
KAVEH	KAYDAN	KAYLEE
KAVEL	KAYDANCE	KAYLEEN
KAVELL	KAYDE	KAYLEI
KAVELLE	KAYDEE	KAYLEIGH
KAVEN	KAYDEE-LEIGH	KAYLEIGH-ANN
KAVI	KAYDEN	KAYLEIGH-ANNE
KAVIN	KAYDEN-JAMES	KAYLEIGH-JANE
KAVINA	KAYDEN-JAY	KAYLEIGH-LOUISE
KAVINAYAN	KAYDEN-JOHN	KAYLEIGH-MARIE
KAVIR	KAYDEN-LEE	KAYLEIGH-MAY
KAVISH	KAYDEN-SCOTT	KAYLEIGH-ROSE
KAVISHA	KAYDENCE	KAYLEM
KAVISHAN	KAYDEY	KAYLEN
KAVISNA	KAYDI	KAYLEY
KAVITA	KAYDI-LEIGH	KAYLI
KAVIYA	KAYDIAN	KAYLIA

KAYLIB
KAYLIE
KAYLIEGH
KAYLIN
KAYLLA
KAYLLUM
KAYLN
KAYLON
KAYLUB
KAYLUM
KAYLUN
KAYLYN
KAYN
KAYNA
KAYNAAT
KAYNAN
KAYNAT
KAYNATH
KAYNE
KAYNEN
KAYO
KAYODE
KAYON
KAYORI
KAYRA
KAYSAAN
KAYSAH
KAYSAN
KAYSEN
KAYSER
KAYSEY
KAYSHA
KAYSHIA
KAYSI
KAYSIE
KAYSON
KAYSON-JAMES
KAYTE
KAYTEE
KAYTI
KAYTIE
KAYTLIN
KAYTLYN
KAYTON
KAYVAN
KAYWAN
KAYYAN
KAYZIA

KAZ
KAZEEM
KAZI
KAZIA
KAZIAH
KAZIM
KAZIMIERZ
KAZUKI
KC
KE
KEA
KEAGAN
KEAH
KEAIRA
KEAL
KEALA
KEALAN
KEALEIGH
KEALEN
KEALEY
KEALIE
KEALY
KEAN
KEANA
KEANAH
KEANAN
KEANDRE
KEANE
KEANEN
KEANNA
KEANNE
KEANO
KEANON
KEANU
KEANUN
KEAON
KEARA
KEARAN
KEAREN
KEARNA
KEARNEY
KEARNO
KEARON
KEASHA
KEATAN
KEATEN
KEATON
KEATON-LEE

KEAUNA
KEAVA
KEAVEY
KEAVIE
KEAVY
KEBBA
KEBRON
KEDUS
KEEAN
KEEDIE
KEEFE
KEEGAN
KEEGAN-LEE
KEEHAN
KEELA
KEELAN
KEELEA
KEELEE
KEELEIGH
KEELEN
KEELEY
KEELEY-ANN
KEELEY-MAE
KEELEY-ROSE
KEELI
KEELIA
KEELIE
KEELIN
KEELY
KEENAN
KEENEN
KEENON
KEERA
KEERAN
KEERAT
KEERATH
KEERIT
KEERON
KEERTAN
KEERTHANA
KEERTHI
KEERTHIKA
KEES
KEESHA
KEETAN
KEETON
KEEVA
KEEVAH

KEEVI
KEEVIE
KEEVY
KEEYA
KEEYAN
KEGAN
KEHARA
KEHINDE
KEHLANI
KEI
KEIA
KEIAN
KEIANA
KEIANNA
KEIARA
KEIARAH
KEIDA
KEIDEN
KEIFER
KEIGAN
KEIGHAN
KEIGHLEY
KEIGHTON
KEIGO
KEIKO
KEIL
KEILA
KEILAH
KEILAN
KEILANA
KEILEIGH
KEILEY
KEILY
KEINAN
KEION
KEIR
KEIRA
KEIRA-LEA
KEIRA-LEE
KEIRA-LEIGH
KEIRA-LOUISE
KEIRA-MAE
KEIRA-MAI
KEIRA-MARIE
KEIRA-MAY
KEIRA-ROSE
KEIRAH
KEIRALEIGH

KEIRAN
KEIREN
KEIRON
KEIRRA
KEIRRAN
KEIRYN
KEISHA
KEISI
KEITA
KEITH
KEITHA
KEITIJA
KEITON
KEIVA
KEIYAN
KEIYONA
KEJAUN
KEJSI
KEKELI
KEL
KELAN
KELBY
KELCEE
KELCEY
KELCI
KELCIE
KELCY
KELDA
KELDON
KELECHI
KELEIGH
KELHAM
KELI
KELIA
KELIS
KELISA
KELISE
KELISHA
KELL
KELLA
KELLAN
KELLAND
KELLE
KELLEN
KELLER
KELLEY
KELLI
KELLIANNE

KELLIE
KELLIE-ANN
KELLIE-MARIE
KELLIN
KELLIS
KELLISE
KELLSEY
KELLSIE
KELLUM
KELLY
KELLY-ANN
KELLY-ANNE
KELLY-JO
KELLY-LOUISE
KELLY-MARIE
KELLYANN
KELLYANNE
KELLYMARIE
KELSA
KELSEA
KELSEE
KELSEI
KELSEIGH
KELSEY
KELSEY-
KELSEY-JO
KELSEY-LEIGH
KELSEY-LOUISE
KELSEY-MAE
KELSEY-MAI
KELSEY-MAY
KELSEY-RAE
KELSI
KELSIE
KELSIE-ANN
KELSIE-LEIGH
KELSIE-MAE
KELSIE-MAI
KELSIE-MARIE
KELSIE-MAY
KELSIE-ROSE
KELSO
KELSON
KELSTON
KELSY
KELTON
KELVIN
KELYAN

KELYN
KEMAL
KEMANI
KEMANIE
KEMAR
KEMARI
KEMI
KEMIYAH
KEMUEL
KEN
KENADIE
KENAI
KENAN
KENAYA
KENAYAH
KENDA
KENDAL
KENDALL
KENDAN
KENDEL
KENDELL
KENDON
KENDRA
KENDRICK
KENDYL
KENECHI
KENECHUKWU
KENEIL
KENENNA
KENIA
KENISHA
KENJI
KENLEE
KENLEY
KENNA
KENNADIE
KENNADY
KENNEDI
KENNEDIE
KENNEDY
KENNETH
KENNIE
KENNY
KENO
KENON
KENRICK
KENSA
KENSEY

KENSHIRO
KENSI
KENSIE
KENSLEY
KENT
KENTARO
KENTO
KENTON
KENYA
KENYA-ROSE
KENYAH
KENYON
KENZA
KENZEE
KENZI
KENZIE
KENZIE-J
KENZIE-JAMES
KENZIE-JAY
KENZIE-LEE
KENZO
KENZY
KEO
KEOGH
KEON
KEONA
KEONE
KEONI
KEOWN
KERA
KERALA
KERAN
KERBY
KEREECE
KEREM
KEREN
KERENA
KERENSA
KERENZA
KERI
KERI-ANN
KERI-ANNE
KERIA
KERIAN
KERIANNE
KERIM
KERIN
KERINA

KERIS
KERISHA
KERISS
KERN
KERNIUS
KERON
KERR
KERRA
KERRI
KERRI-ANN
KERRI-ANNE
KERRIANN
KERRIANNE
KERRIE
KERRIE-ANN
KERRIE-ANNE
KERRIGAN
KERRIN
KERRIS
KERRON
KERRY
KERRY-ANN
KERRY-ANNE
KERRY-LEE
KERRY-LEIGH
KERRY-LOUISE
KERRYANN
KERRYANNE
KERRYN
KERSHA
KERSTIN
KERVIN
KERYN
KERYS
KES
KESAR
KESAVAN
KESHA
KESHAN
KESHAUN
KESHAV
KESHAVA
KESHAVI
KESHAWN
KESHET
KESHIA
KESHIKA
KESHINI

KESHNI
KESHVI
KESIA
KESIENA
KESLEY
KESSER
KESSIA
KESSIE
KESTER
KESTON
KESTRA
KETAN
KETIA
KETIJA
KETRIN
KETSIA
KETURAH
KETZIAH
KEVA
KEVAL
KEVAN
KEVELL
KEVELLE
KEVEN
KEVIN
KEVINA
KEVINAS
KEVINS
KEVON
KEVSER
KEWAN
KEWELL
KEWIN
KEXIN
KEYA
KEYAAN
KEYAH
KEYAN
KEYANA
KEYANNA
KEYARA
KEYARNA
KEYLA
KEYLAN
KEYLEE
KEYLEIGH
KEYLEY
KEYON
KEYON'DRE
KEYONTE
KEYRA
KEYSHA
KEYSHAWN
KEYSHIA
KEZ
KEZI
KEZIA
KEZIAH
KEZZIA
KHAALID
KHADAR
KHADEEJA
KHADEEJAH
KHADEEM
KHADEJA
KHADEJAH
KHADEJIA
KHADEZA
KHADIDJA
KHADIGA
KHADIIJA
KHADIJA
KHADIJAH
KHADIJAT
KHADIJHA
KHADIJO
KHADIM
KHADIZA
KHADIZAH
KHADRA
KHAI
KHAILA
KHAIRA
KHAIRAH
KHAIRO
KHAIRUL
KHAIRUN
KHALAM
KHALEB
KHALED
KHALEDA
KHALEED
KHALEEL
KHALEEM
KHALEEQ
KHALEEQA
KHALEESAH
KHALEESI
KHALEL
KHALEN
KHALI
KHALIA
KHALIAH
KHALID
KHALIDA
KHALIDAH
KHALIF
KHALIFA
KHALIFAH
KHALIL
KHALILA
KHALILAH
KHALIM
KHALIQ
KHALIS
KHALISA
KHALISAH
KHALISHA
KHALIYA
KHALIYAH
KHAMAL
KHAMANI
KHAMARI
KHAMARNI
KHAN
KHANDAKER
KHANDOKAR
KHANG
KHANH
KHANSA
KHANSAA
KHANYA
KHANYISILE
KHAQAN
KHARA
KHARI
KHARIS
KHASHIF
KHATEEB
KHATIJA
KHATIJAH
KHATTAB
KHAULAH
KHAVAR

KHAWAJA
KHAWAR
KHAWLA
KHAWLAH
KHAYA
KHAYAL
KHAYAM
KHAYAN
KHAYDEN
KHAYLA
KHAYLEN
KHAYRA
KHAYRAH
KHAYRI
KHAYYAM
KHAZEEMA
KHEA
KHEIRA
KHEM
KHEZAR
KHI
KHIA
KHIAH
KHIAN
KHIANA
KHIANNA
KHIARA
KHIRA
KHIRAD
KHIVI
KHIYA
KHIYAN
KHIZAR
KHIZER
KHIZR
KHIZRA
KHLOE
KHLOEY
KHODI
KHOLA
KHOURTNEY
KHRISH
KHRISHA
KHRISTIAN
KHUBAIB
KHUBAYB
KHULAN
KHULUD

KHURAM
KHURRAM
KHURUM
KHUSBU
KHUSH
KHUSHAL
KHUSHALI
KHUSHBOO
KHUSHBU
KHUSHI
KHUSHPREET
KHUSI
KHUZAYMAH
KHWAISH
KHWAJA
KHY
KHYA
KHYAN
KHYANNA
KHYATI
KHYBER
KHYE
KHYLA
KHYLAN
KHYLE
KHYRA
KHYRAN
KHYREE
KHYREN
KHYRON
KI
KIA
KIA-LEIGH
KIA-LOUISE
KIA-MAI
KIA-MARIE
KIA-ROSE
KIAAN
KIAH
KIAHNA
KIAL
KIALL
KIAM
KIAN
KIAN-JAMES
KIAN-JAY
KIAN-LEE
KIANA

KIANAH
KIANE
KIANI
KIANNA
KIANNA-ROSE
KIANNAH
KIANNE
KIANO
KIAO
KIARA
KIARA-LEIGH
KIARA-MAY
KIARAH
KIARAN
KIARASH
KIARN
KIARNA
KIARNO
KIARON
KIARRA
KIARRAH
KIAS
KIAYA
KIDA
KIDUS
KIE
KIEAN
KIEANA
KIEANNA
KIEARA
KIEARNA
KIEDIS
KIEFER
KIEFFER
KIEGAN
KIEL
KIELA
KIELAN
KIEN
KIENAN
KIENNA
KIEON
KIER
KIERA
KIERA-LEIGH
KIERA-LOUISE
KIERA-MAE
KIERA-MAY

KIERA-ROSE	KIMON	KIRANVEER
KIERAH	KIMORA	KIRAT
KIERAN	KIMORA-LEE	KIRBIE
KIERAN-LEE	KIMRAN	KIRBY
KIERANLEE	KIN	KIREAN
KIERAT	KINAAN	KIREN
KIEREN	KINAN	KIRENDEEP
KIERIAN	KINCSO	KIRI
KIERNAN	KINDA	KIRIL
KIERON	KING	KIRILL
KIERON-LEE	KING-DAVID	KIRILLS
KIERRA	KINGA	KIRILS
KIERRAN	KINGDAVID	KIRIN
KIERREN	KINGSLEIGH	KIRIT
KIERRON	KINGSLEY	KIRK
KIERSTEN	KINGSON	KIRO
KIERYN	KINGSTON	KIRON
KIESHA	KINJAL	KIRPA
KIETAN	KINLEE	KIRPAL
KIEVA	KINLEY	KIRRA
KIKA	KINNARI	KIRRAN
KIKELOMO	KINSEY	KIRREN
KIKI	KINSLEY	KIRSTEN
KIKO	KINVARA	KIRSTEY
KILA	KINZA	KIRSTI
KILE	KINZAH	KIRSTIE
KILIAN	KIO	KIRSTIN
KILLIAN	KIOMI	KIRSTINA
KIM	KION	KIRSTY
KIMAN	KIONA	KIRSTY-ANN
KIMANI	KIONI	KIRSTY-JANE
KIMARA	KIP	KIRSTY-LOUISE
KIMARLEY	KIPP	KIRSTY-MARIE
KIMARNI	KIPRAS	KIRSTYN
KIMAYA	KIRA	KIRTAN
KIMBALL	KIRA-LEIGH	KIRTHANA
KIMBERLEE	KIRA-NERYS	KIRTHIKA
KIMBERLEIGH	KIRA-ROSE	KIRTI
KIMBERLEY	KIRAH	KIRTIS
KIMBERLEY-JO	KIRAN	KIRUBEL
KIMBERLIE	KIRANA	KIRUTHIK
KIMBERLY	KIRANDEEP	KIRUTHIKA
KIMI	KIRANDIP	KISA
KIMIA	KIRANI	KISAN
KIMIKO	KIRANJEET	KISANET
KIMIYA	KIRANJIT	KISHA
KIMMI	KIRANJOT	KISHAAN
KIMMY	KIRANPREET	KISHAN

KISHANA	KLARISSA	KODA
KISHANI	KLAUDIA	KODEE
KISHEN	KLAUDIE	KODEN
KISHI	KLAUDIJA	KODEY
KISHON	KLAUDIJUS	KODI
KISHOR	KLAUDIO	KODIE
KISHORE	KLAUDIUSZ	KODY
KISHWAR	KLAUS	KODY-LEE
KISMAT	KLAVS	KOEN
KISMET	KLAY	KOFI
KISWA	KLAYTON	KOHAN
KISWAH	KLEA	KOHANA
KIT	KLEART	KOHEI
KITA	KLEDI	KOHEN
KITAI	KLEIN	KOHINOOR
KITANA	KLEIO	KOHKI
KITO	KLEO	KOHL
KITSON	KLEON	KOI
KITT	KLEOPATRA	KOJI
KITTI	KLESTI	KOJO
KITTIE	KLEVIS	KOKI
KITTO	KLEVISA	KOKO
KITTY	KLINE	KOLADE
KITTY-ROSE	KLODIAN	KOLAWOLE
KIVA	KLOE	KOLBE
KIVANC	KLYNE	KOLBI
KIY	KNIGHT	KOLBIE
KIYA	KNOX	KOLBY
KIYAAN	KOA	KOLE
KIYAH	KOAH	KOLI
KIYAN	KOAN	KOLOS
KIYANA	KOBAN	KOLSUMA
KIYANI	KOBBY	KOLTON
KIYANNA	KOBE	KOMAL
KIYANSH	KOBEE	KOMALPREET
KIYARA	KOBEN	KONA
KIYARNA	KOBEY	KONAIN
KIYLA	KOBEY-JAMES	KONAN
KIYOMI	KOBI	KONDRAD
KIYON	KOBI-JAMES	KONNA
KIYRA	KOBI-JAY	KONNAH
KIZZI	KOBIE	KONNAR
KIZZIE	KOBIE-LEE	KONNER
KIZZY	KOBINA	KONNIE
KLAIDAS	KOBURN	KONNOR
KLAIDI	KOBY	KONOR
KLAJDI	KOBY-LEE	KONRAD
KLARA	KOBYN	KONSTANTIN

KONSTANTINA	KOURTNIE	KRISTIEN
KONSTANTINE	KOUSHIK	KRISTIN
KONSTANTINOS	KOVAN	KRISTINA
KONSTANTY	KOWSAR	KRISTINE
KOOPER	KOYUKI	KRISTIYAN
KORA	KRAIG	KRISTIYANA
KORAH	KRASIMIR	KRISTJAN
KORAL	KRAY	KRISTOF
KORAN	KRINA	KRISTOFER
KORAY	KRIPA	KRISTOFERS
KORBAN	KRIS	KRISTOFF
KORBEN	KRISH	KRISTOFFER
KORBIN	KRISHA	KRISTON
KORBON	KRISHAN	KRISTOPHER
KORBY	KRISHANG	KRISTOS
KORBYN	KRISHANTH	KRISTUPAS
KORDEL	KRISHAV	KRISTY
KORDELIA	KRISHAY	KRISTYN
KORDELL	KRISHEN	KRISTYNA
KORDIAN	KRISHI	KRISZTIAN
KOREDE	KRISHIKA	KRIT
KOREN	KRISHIV	KRITHIK
KOREY	KRISHMA	KRITHIKA
KOREY-LEE	KRISHNA	KRITI
KORI	KRISHNAN	KRITIKA
KORIE	KRISHNI	KRITTIKA
KORIN	KRISHTI	KRIYA
KORINA	KRISIA	KRON
KORNEL	KRISIYA	KRRISH
KORNELIA	KRISMA	KRUM
KORNELIJA	KRISS	KRUPA
KORNELIJUS	KRISSIE	KRUZ
KORNELIUSZ	KRISSY	KRUZE
KORRA	KRISTA	KRYSPIN
KORRI	KRISTAL	KRYSTA
KORRIE	KRISTAN	KRYSTAL
KORTNEY	KRISTAPS	KRYSTAL-ROSE
KORY	KRISTEL	KRYSTEL
KORYN	KRISTELLE	KRYSTEN
KOSHAN	KRISTEN	KRYSTIAN
KOSISOCHUKWU	KRISTERS	KRYSTINA
KOSMA	KRISTI	KRYSTLE
KOSTA	KRISTIA	KRYSTOF
KOSTAS	KRISTIAAN	KRYSTYNA
KOTA	KRISTIAN	KRZYSZTOF
KOTRYNA	KRISTIANA	KSAWERY
KOUROSH	KRISTIANS	KSAWIER
KOURTNEY	KRISTIE	KSENIA

KSENIJA
KSENIYA
KSHAF
KT
KUBA
KUBILAY
KUBRA
KUBRAH
KUDAKWASHE
KUDUS
KUDZAI
KULDIP
KULJEET
KULJIT
KULRAJ
KULREET
KULSOOM
KULSUM
KULSUMA
KULTHOOM
KULTHUM
KULVEER
KUMAIL
KUMAR
KUMARAN
KUMARI
KUMAYL
KUMBA
KUN
KUNAAL
KUNAL
KUNASHE
KUNDAI
KUNJ
KUNWAR
KUPAKWASHE
KUPRA
KURAN
KURRAN
KURT
KURTIS
KURTISS
KURUN
KUSH
KUSHAGRA
KUSHAL
KUSHI
KUZEY

KUZIVA
KWABENA
KWADWO
KWAJO
KWAKU
KWAME
KWASI
KWEKU
KWESI
KWOK
KY
KY-MANI
KY'MANI
KYA
KYAAN
KYAH
KYAL
KYALL
KYAN
KYANA
KYANN
KYANNA
KYANNE
KYARA
KYARNA
KYAS
KYDAN
KYDEN
KYDON
KYE
KYE-JAMES
KYEA
KYEDEN
KYEISHA
KYEL
KYELAN
KYELL
KYEN
KYERAN
KYERON
KYESHA
KYI
KYIA
KYIAH
KYIAN
KYISHA
KYLA
KYLA-JADE

KYLA-JO
KYLA-LEIGH
KYLA-MAE
KYLA-MAI
KYLA-MAY
KYLA-RAE
KYLA-ROSE
KYLAH
KYLAH-ROSE
KYLAN
KYLAN-JAI
KYLAR
KYLE
KYLE-JUNIOR
KYLEN
KYLER
KYLIAN
KYLIE
KYLO
KYLON
KYLUM
KYLUN
KYM
KYMANI
KYMARA
KYMARI
KYMARNI
KYMBERLEY
KYMBERLY
KYMORA
KYMRAN
KYNA
KYNAAT
KYNAN
KYO
KYOKO
KYOMI
KYOMIE
KYON
KYPROS
KYRA
KYRA-LEA
KYRA-LEIGH
KYRA-LOUISE
KYRA-MAE
KYRA-MAI
KYRA-MAY
KYRA-ROSE

KYRAH
KYRAH-LEIGH
KYRALEIGH
KYRAN
KYRAN-JAMES
KYRAN-LEE
KYRECE
KYREE
KYREECE
KYREESE
KYREL
KYRELL
KYRELLE
KYREN
KYRENE
KYRESE
KYRHYS
KYRI
KYRIA
KYRIACOS
KYRIAKI
KYRIAKOS
KYRIAN
KYRIE
KYRIQUE
KYRO
KYRON
KYRON-JAMES
KYRON-LEE
KYRONE
KYROS
KYRUN
KYRUS
KYSON
KYTE
KYU
KYZA
KYZER

L

L	LACEY-KAY	LAELA
L-JAY	LACEY-LEA	LAELIA
L'MAR	LACEY-LEE	LAETICIA
L'RAE	LACEY-LEIGH	LAETITIA
L'SHAE	LACEY-LOU	LAGAN
L'WREN	LACEY-LOUISE	LAGERTHA
LA	LACEY-MAE	LAHAN
LA-ROSA	LACEY-MAI	LAHNA
LA'	LACEY-MARIE	LAHNI
LA'KAI	LACEY-MAY	LAI
LA'RAE	LACEY-MAYE	LAIA
LA'TIA	LACEY-RAE	LAIBA
LAAIBA	LACEY-RAI	LAIBAA
LAAIBAH	LACEY-ROSE	LAIBAAH
LAAIQAH	LACEY-SUMMER	LAIBAH
LAANA	LACEYMAE	LAICE
LAARNI	LACEYMAY	LAICEE
LAASYA	LACHEZAR	LAICEY
LABAN	LACHLAN	LAICIE
LABEEB	LACHLANN	LAIGAN
LABEEBA	LACI	LAIGHTON
LABEEBAH	LACI-MAE	LAIHA
LABEENA	LACI-MAI	LAIKA
LABEEQA	LACIE	LAIKE
LABIB	LACIE-ANN	LAIKEN
LABIBA	LACIE-ANNE	LAILA
LABIBAH	LACIE-JAI	LAILA-GRACE
LACE	LACIE-JANE	LAILA-MAE
LACEE	LACIE-JAYNE	LAILA-MAI
LACEE-MAE	LACIE-LEIGH	LAILA-MARIE
LACEIGH	LACIE-LOU	LAILA-MAY
LACEY	LACIE-LOUISE	LAILA-RAE
LACEY-	LACIE-MAE	LAILA-ROSE
LACEY-ANN	LACIE-MAI	LAILAA
LACEY-ANNE	LACIE-MARIE	LAILAH
LACEY-DEE	LACIE-MAY	LAILAND
LACEY-GRACE	LACIE-RAE	LAILY
LACEY-JADE	LACIE-ROSE	LAIMA
LACEY-JAE	LACIEE	LAINA
LACEY-JAI	LACY	LAINE
LACEY-JANE	LACY-MAE	LAINEE
LACEY-JAY	LACY-MAY	LAINEY
LACEY-JAYNE	LADA	LAINEY-RAE
LACEY-JO	LADAN	LAINI
	LADINA	LAINIE
	LADISLAV	LAINNIE
	LADY	LAINY
	LAEL	LAIQA

LAIQAH
LAIRA
LAIRD
LAISHA
LAISON
LAITEN
LAITH
LAITHAN
LAITON
LAITYN
LAIYA
LAIYAH
LAIYBA
LAIYLA
LAKAI
LAKAYA
LAKE
LAKEISHA
LAKEIYA
LAKELAN
LAKEN
LAKESHA
LAKHAI
LAKHAN
LAKHVEER
LAKHVINDER
LAKIESHA
LAKISHA
LAKITA
LAKOTA
LAKSH
LAKSHA
LAKSHAN
LAKSHANA
LAKSHAY
LAKSHMAN
LAKSHMI
LAKSHYA
LALANA
LALE
LALI
LALITA
LALITHA
LALO
LAM
LAMA
LAMAAR
LAMAISAH

LAMAR
LAMARA
LAMARI
LAMARR
LAMBROS
LAMEES
LAMEESAH
LAMEK
LAMIA
LAMIAH
LAMIN
LAMINE
LAMIS
LAMISA
LAMISAH
LAMISHA
LAMIYA
LAMIYAH
LAMONT
LAMORNA
LAMYA
LAN
LANA
LANA-MAE
LANA-MAY
LANA-ROSE
LANAE
LANAH
LANAI
LANAIS
LANAYA
LANCE
LANCELOT
LANDEN
LANDER
LANDO
LANDON
LANE
LANELLE
LANEY
LANI
LANIA
LANIE
LANIKA
LANIYA
LANIYAH
LANNA
LANO

LANRE
LANY
LANYA
LANZ
LAOISE
LAQUAN
LAQUISHA
LAQUITA
LARA
LARA-JADE
LARA-MAE
LARA-MAY
LARA-ROSE
LARAE
LARAH
LARAIB
LARANYA
LARAYA
LARAYAH
LARAYB
LAREB
LAREEN
LARELL
LAREN
LARENA
LARENZ
LARENZO
LARIA
LARIAH
LARIN
LARISA
LARISSA
LARIYA
LARK
LARKIN
LARNA
LARNI
LARNIE
LAROSA
LARRISSA
LARRY
LARS
LARSON
LARSSON
LARYSA
LARYSSA
LAS
LASHA

LASHAE	LATOYA	LAURYNAS
LASHAI	LATOYAH	LAVA
LASHAN	LATRELL	LAVAN
LASHANA	LATRELLE	LAVAND
LASHANNA	LAUCHLAN	LAVANYA
LASHARN	LAUMA	LAVAYAH
LASHARNA	LAUNA	LAVEAH
LASHARNE	LAURA	LAVEEN
LASHAWN	LAURA-	LAVEEZA
LASHAY	LAURA-ANN	LAVELL
LASHAYA	LAURA-ANNE	LAVELLE
LASON	LAURA-BETH	LAVENDER
LASSANA	LAURA-JANE	LAVERNE
LASYA	LAURA-JAYNE	LAVIA
LASZLO	LAURA-JO	LAVIN
LATALIA	LAURA-LOUISE	LAVINA
LATANYA	LAURA-MAY	LAVINIA
LATASHA	LAURA-ROSE	LAVINYA
LATASIA	LAURAN	LAW
LATAYA	LAURANCE	LAWA
LATAYAH	LAURE	LAWAN
LATEEF	LAUREEN	LAWAND
LATEEFA	LAUREL	LAWE
LATEEFAH	LAURELL	LAWEE
LATEEFAT	LAURELLE	LAWEN
LATEEN	LAUREN	LAWI
LATEESHA	LAUREN-JADE	LAWIE
LATEISHA	LAUREN-LOUISE	LAWIN
LATESHA	LAUREN-MAE	LAWRANCE
LATHAM	LAUREN-MARIE	LAWREN
LATHAN	LAUREN-ROSE	LAWRENCE
LATHANIEL	LAURENA	LAWRIE
LATHEN	LAURENCE	LAWSON
LATHUSAN	LAURENE	LAWTON
LATHUSHAN	LAURENNE	LAWY
LATIA	LAURENS	LAXMAN
LATICIA	LAURENT	LAXMI
LATIF	LAURENTIU	LAXMITHA
LATIFA	LAURETTA	LAXSHAN
LATIFAH	LAURI	LAYA
LATIFAT	LAURIANNE	LAYAAL
LATIKA	LAURICE	LAYAAN
LATIN	LAURIE	LAYAD
LATINA	LAURIE-ANNE	LAYAH
LATISHA	LAURIS	LAYAL
LATITIA	LAURISSA	LAYALI
LATIYA	LAURREN	LAYAN
LATONIA	LAURYN	LAYANA

LAYANAH
LAYANNE
LAYBA
LAYBAH
LAYCEE
LAYCEE-MAE
LAYCEY
LAYCI
LAYCIE
LAYDEN
LAYKE
LAYKEN
LAYLA
LAYLA-ANN
LAYLA-ANNE
LAYLA-BEAU
LAYLA-BELLE
LAYLA-FAYE
LAYLA-GRACE
LAYLA-JADE
LAYLA-JAI
LAYLA-JANE
LAYLA-JAY
LAYLA-JAYNE
LAYLA-JEAN
LAYLA-LEIGH
LAYLA-LOUISE
LAYLA-MAE
LAYLA-MAI
LAYLA-MARIE
LAYLA-MAY
LAYLA-RAE
LAYLA-ROSE
LAYLAA
LAYLAH
LAYLAH-ROSE
LAYLAN
LAYLAND
LAYLANI
LAYLEN
LAYLI
LAYLIE
LAYLON
LAYNA
LAYNE
LAYNEE
LAYNI
LAYNIE
LAYSON
LAYTAN
LAYTEN
LAYTH
LAYTHAM
LAYTHAN
LAYTON
LAYTON-JAMES
LAYTON-JAY
LAYTON-JOHN
LAYTON-LEE
LAYYAH
LAYYANAH
LAYYINAH
LAZAR
LAZARUS
LAZER
LAZO
LE
LE-ANN
LEA
LEA-MARIE
LEAH
LEAH-ANN
LEAH-GRACE
LEAH-JADE
LEAH-JANE
LEAH-JAYNE
LEAH-LOUISE
LEAH-MAE
LEAH-MAI
LEAH-MARIE
LEAH-MAY
LEAH-PAIGE
LEAH-ROSE
LEAHA
LEALA
LEALAN
LEALAND
LEAM
LEANA
LEANAH
LEANDA
LEANDER
LEANDRA
LEANDRE
LEANDRO
LEANDROS
LEANE
LEANN
LEANNA
LEANNAH
LEANNE
LEANOR
LEANORA
LEARA
LEARNA
LEART
LEASHA
LEATITIA
LEAYA
LEBAN
LEBRON
LEDA
LEDIANA
LEDIO
LEDION
LEDJON
LEDLEY
LEE
LEE-ANN
LEE-ANNE
LEE-JAMES
LEE-JAY
LEE-JUNIOR
LEEA
LEEAH
LEEAM
LEEANN
LEEANNA
LEEANNE
LEEBAN
LEEGAN
LEEJAY
LEELA
LEELA-MAE
LEELA-ROSE
LEELAH
LEELAN
LEELAND
LEELOO
LEEMA
LEEN
LEENA
LEENAH
LEEON

LEEROY	LEILAH-MAE	LENKA
LEESA	LEILAN	LENNA
LEESHA	LEILAND	LENNAN
LEESON	LEILANI	LENNARD
LEEVI	LEILIA	LENNART
LEEYA	LEINA	LENNI
LEEYAH	LEIRE	LENNIE
LEEZA	LEISA	LENNIX
LEGEND	LEISHA	LENNON
LEHA	LEITH	LENNOX
LEHAT	LEIYA	LENNY
LEI	LEIYAH	LENNY-JOE
LEIA	LEJA	LENON
LEIA-ROSE	LEJLA	LENORA
LEIAH	LEKAI	LENORE
LEIAM	LEKEISHA	LENOX
LEIANA	LEKISHA	LENY
LEIANNA	LELA	LENYA
LEIARNA	LELAH	LEO
LEIF	LELAINA	LEO-JAI
LEIGH	LELAN	LEO-JAMES
LEIGH-ANN	LELAND	LEO-JAY
LEIGH-ANNA	LELAND-JAMES	LEO-JOHN
LEIGH-ANNE	LELANI	LEO-RILEY
LEIGHA	LELIA	LEOLA
LEIGHA-LOUISE	LELIANA	LEOM
LEIGHAH	LELIE	LEON
LEIGHAM	LEMA	LEON-JAMES
LEIGHANN	LEMAR	LEON-JUNIOR
LEIGHANNA	LEMARI	LEONA
LEIGHANNE	LEMARR	LEONAH
LEIGHARNA	LEMMY	LEONARD
LEIGHLA	LEMUEL	LEONARDA
LEIGHLAN	LEMUELLA	LEONARDAS
LEIGHLAND	LEN	LEONARDO
LEIGHTON	LENA	LEONARDS
LEIGHTON-JAMES	LENA-MARIE	LEONAS
LEIGHTON-LEE	LENAE	LEONDRE
LEIHA	LENAH	LEONE
LEILA	LENARD	LEONEL
LEILA-GRACE	LENAY	LEONELA
LEILA-MAE	LENAYA	LEONELL
LEILA-MAI	LENAYAH	LEONHARD
LEILA-MARIE	LENE	LEONI
LEILA-MAY	LENI	LEONI-MAY
LEILA-RAE	LENIA	LEONID
LEILA-ROSE	LENINA	LEONIDAS
LEILAH	LENISHA	LEONIDES

LEONIE	LEV	LEXI-JAE
LEONIS	LEVAEH	LEXI-JAI
LEONIT	LEVAN	LEXI-JANE
LEONNA	LEVANA	LEXI-JAY
LEONNE	LEVAYAH	LEXI-JAYNE
LEONNI	LEVEN	LEXI-JEAN
LEONNIE	LEVENT	LEXI-JO
LEONOR	LEVENTE	LEXI-LEA
LEONORA	LEVI	LEXI-LEE
LEONORE	LEVI-JAMES	LEXI-LEI
LEONY	LEVI-JAY	LEXI-LEIGH
LEOPOLD	LEVIE	LEXI-LOU
LEORA	LEVII	LEXI-LOUISE
LEOS	LEVIN	LEXI-MAE
LEOTRIM	LEVINA	LEXI-MAI
LERA	LEVISON	LEXI-MARIE
LERATO	LEVON	LEXI-MAY
LERON	LEVY	LEXI-PAIGE
LERONE	LEWA	LEXI-RAE
LEROY	LEWAN	LEXI-ROSE
LERRYN	LEWEN	LEXI-SKYE
LES	LEWES	LEXIA
LESEDI	LEWEY	LEXIE
LESHAE	LEWI	LEXIE-
LESHAY	LEWIE	LEXIE-ANN
LESLEY	LEWIN	LEXIE-ANNE
LESLEY-ANNE	LEWIS	LEXIE-GRACE
LESLIE	LEWIS-JAMES	LEXIE-JADE
LESTER	LEWIS-JAY	LEXIE-JANE
LETEISHA	LEWIS-JOHN	LEXIE-JAY
LETESHA	LEWIS-JUNIOR	LEXIE-JAYNE
LETIA	LEWIS-LEE	LEXIE-JO
LETICIA	LEWISS	LEXIE-LEIGH
LETICIJA	LEWY	LEXIE-LOU
LETISHA	LEWYN	LEXIE-LOUISE
LETISIA	LEWYS	LEXIE-MAE
LETITIA	LEX	LEXIE-MAI
LETIZIA	LEXA	LEXIE-MARIE
LETO	LEXCI	LEXIE-MAY
LETRELL	LEXEY	LEXIE-RAE
LETTI	LEXI	LEXIE-ROSE
LETTICE	LEXI-	LEXII
LETTIE	LEXI-ANN	LEXII-MAE
LETTY	LEXI-ANNE	LEXII-MAY
LEUAN	LEXI-ELISE	LEXILEIGH
LEUL	LEXI-GRACE	LEXINE
LEUSA	LEXI-J	LEXIS
LEUTRIM	LEXI-JADE	LEXON

LEXSIE	LIARNA	LIIBAAN
LEXTON	LIAS	LIIBAN
LEXUS	LIAT	LIJA
LEXX	LIBA	LIJAH
LEXXI	LIBAAN	LIJANA
LEXXIE	LIBAH	LIL
LEXY	LIBAN	LILA
LEYA	LIBBEY	LILA-GRACE
LEYAH	LIBBI	LILA-MAE
LEYAN	LIBBIE	LILA-ROSE
LEYANA	LIBBIE-MAE	LILAC
LEYANNA	LIBBY	LILAH
LEYLA	LIBBY-	LILAH-GRACE
LEYLA-MAE	LIBBY-ANN	LILAH-MAE
LEYLA-MAY	LIBBY-ANNE	LILAH-MAI
LEYLA-ROSE	LIBBY-GRACE	LILAH-MAY
LEYLAH	LIBBY-JANE	LILAH-RAE
LEYLAN	LIBBY-JO	LILAH-ROSE
LEYLAND	LIBBY-LEIGH	LILANI
LEYLI	LIBBY-LOUISE	LILE
LEYNA	LIBBY-MAE	LILEE
LEYO	LIBBY-MAI	LILEIGH
LEYON	LIBBY-MARIE	LILI
LEYTON	LIBBY-MAY	LILI-ANN
LEZMA	LIBBY-RAE	LILI-ELLA
LI	LIBBY-ROSE	LILI-GRACE
LIA	LIBERTIE	LILI-HAF
LIA-MARIE	LIBERTY	LILI-MAE
LIA-ROSE	LIBERTY-GRACE	LILI-MAI
LIABA	LIBERTY-MAE	LILI-MAY
LIABAH	LIBERTY-ROSE	LILI-ROSE
LIAH	LIBI	LILIA
LIAHONA	LIBIN	LILIA-MAE
LIALA	LIBY	LILIA-ROSE
LIAM	LICIA	LILIAH
LIAM-JAMES	LIDA	LILIAN
LIAM-JAY	LIDIA	LILIAN-ROSE
LIAM-JUNIOR	LIDYA	LILIANA
LIAN	LIEF	LILIANA-ROSE
LIANA	LIELA	LILIANE
LIANAH	LIELLE	LILIANNA
LIANE	LIEM	LILIANNE
LIANG	LIENNA	LILIBET
LIANI	LIEPA	LILIBETH
LIANIE	LIESEL	LILIE
LIANNA	LIESL	LILIE-MAE
LIANNE	LIEV	LILIELLA
LIARA	LIGIA	LILIEN

LILIJA
LILIJANA
LILIMAE
LILIMAI
LILIMAY
LILIROSE
LILITH
LILIWEN
LILIYA
LILJA
LILJANA
LILLA
LILLAH
LILLANI
LILLE
LILLEE
LILLEE-MAE
LILLEIGH
LILLEY
LILLEY-MAE
LILLEY-MAY
LILLEY-ROSE
LILLI
LILLI-ANN
LILLI-ANNE
LILLI-ELLA
LILLI-GRACE
LILLI-MAE
LILLI-MAI
LILLI-MAY
LILLI-RAE
LILLI-ROSE
LILLIA
LILLIA-ROSE
LILLIAH
LILLIAN
LILLIANA
LILLIANNA
LILLIANNE
LILLIARNA
LILLIBETH
LILLIE
LILLIE-
LILLIE-ANN
LILLIE-ANNA
LILLIE-ANNE
LILLIE-BELLE
LILLIE-ELLA

LILLIE-GRACE
LILLIE-JAI
LILLIE-JANE
LILLIE-JAYNE
LILLIE-JEAN
LILLIE-JO
LILLIE-LOUISE
LILLIE-MAE
LILLIE-MAI
LILLIE-MARIE
LILLIE-MAY
LILLIE-PAIGE
LILLIE-RAE
LILLIE-ROSE
LILLIELLA
LILLIEMAE
LILLIEMAI
LILLIEMAY
LILLIEROSE
LILLIMAE
LILLIMAI
LILLIMAY
LILLIROSE
LILLITH
LILLY
LILLY-
LILLY-ANN
LILLY-ANNA
LILLY-ANNE
LILLY-BEAU
LILLY-BELLE
LILLY-BETH
LILLY-BOW
LILLY-ELLA
LILLY-FAYE
LILLY-GRACE
LILLY-JADE
LILLY-JANE
LILLY-JAYNE
LILLY-JEAN
LILLY-JO
LILLY-LOUISE
LILLY-MAE
LILLY-MAI
LILLY-MARIE
LILLY-MAY
LILLY-PAIGE
LILLY-RAE

LILLY-RAY
LILLY-ROSE
LILLY-SUE
LILLYA
LILLYAN
LILLYANA
LILLYANN
LILLYANNA
LILLYANNE
LILLYARNA
LILLYBELLE
LILLYELLA
LILLYGRACE
LILLYMAE
LILLYMAI
LILLYMAY
LILLYROSE
LILO
LILOU
LILU
LILWEN
LILY
LILY-
LILY-ANN
LILY-ANNA
LILY-ANNE
LILY-BEAU
LILY-BELLE
LILY-BETH
LILY-BO
LILY-ELLA
LILY-EVE
LILY-FAITH
LILY-FAYE
LILY-GRACE
LILY-HOPE
LILY-JADE
LILY-JANE
LILY-JAY
LILY-JAYNE
LILY-JEAN
LILY-JO
LILY-JOY
LILY-KATE
LILY-LEE
LILY-LOUISE
LILY-MAE
LILY-MAI

LILY-MARIE
LILY-MAY
LILY-MAYE
LILY-PAIGE
LILY-RAE
LILY-RAI
LILY-ROSE
LILY-SUE
LILYA
LILYAH
LILYAN
LILYANA
LILYANN
LILYANNA
LILYANNE
LILYBELLE
LILYBETH
LILYELLA
LILYMAE
LILYMAY
LILYROSE
LIMA
LIMARA
LIN
LINA
LINAH
LINARDS
LINAS
LINCOLN
LINCOLN-JAMES
LINCOLN-JAY
LINCON
LINDA
LINDA-MARIE
LINDAN
LINDEN
LINDON
LINDSAY
LINDSEY
LINDY
LINETTE
LINEYSHA
LINFORD
LING
LINH
LINK
LINKIN
LINKOLN

LINKON
LINNEA
LINNET
LINO
LINSEY
LINTON
LINUS
LINXI
LINZI
LIO
LION
LIONA
LIONEL
LIOR
LIORA
LIPA
LIR
LIRA
LIRAN
LIRIM
LIS
LISA
LISA-MARIE
LISAMARIE
LISBETH
LISE
LISETTE
LISHA
LISHANA
LISHANI
LISSA
LISSI
LISSIA
LISSIE
LISSY
LISTON
LITA
LITIA
LITISHA
LIUTAURAS
LIV
LIVA
LIVI
LIVIA
LIVIAH
LIVIANA
LIVIE
LIVIJA

LIVINIA
LIVIO
LIVIU
LIVIYA
LIVLEEN
LIVVI
LIVVIE
LIVVY
LIVY
LIWIA
LIWSI
LIYA
LIYAA
LIYAANA
LIYAANAH
LIYAH
LIYAN
LIYANA
LIYANAH
LIYANNA
LIYARA
LIYBA
LIYBAH
LIYLA
LIYLAH
LIZ
LIZA
LIZE
LIZZI
LIZZIE
LIZZY
LJ
LJAY
LJILJANA
LLANA
LLAYTON
LLEU
LLEUCU
LLEW
LLEWELLYN
LLEWELYN
LLEWYN
LLEYTON
LLIAM
LLIAN
LLIFON
LLINOS
LLIO

LLION
LLIWEN
LLOYD
LLWYD
LLYR
LLYWELYN
LMAR
LOAY
LOCHAN
LOCHIE
LOCHLAIN
LOCHLAINN
LOCHLAN
LOCHLANN
LOCHLEN
LOCHLYN
LOCKE
LOCKIE
LOCKLAN
LOCKLEN
LOCKLYN
LOCRYN
LOEN
LOGAN
LOGAN-JACK
LOGAN-JAI
LOGAN-JAMES
LOGAN-JAY
LOGAN-JOHN
LOGAN-KAI
LOGAN-LEE
LOGAN-REECE
LOGAN-THOMAS
LOGEN
LOGHAN
LOGON
LOGUN
LOHAN
LOHITH
LOHLA
LOIC
LOIS
LOJAIN
LOK
LOKESH
LOKI
LOLA
LOLA-

LOLA-ANNE
LOLA-BELLE
LOLA-BLU
LOLA-BROOKE
LOLA-FAITH
LOLA-GRACE
LOLA-JADE
LOLA-JAI
LOLA-JANE
LOLA-JAY
LOLA-JAYNE
LOLA-JEAN
LOLA-JO
LOLA-LEIGH
LOLA-LOUISE
LOLA-MAE
LOLA-MAI
LOLA-MARIE
LOLA-MAY
LOLA-MIA
LOLA-RAE
LOLA-ROSE
LOLA-SUE
LOLADE
LOLAH
LOLITA
LOLLA
LOLLIE
LOLLY
LOMAX
LONA
LONAN
LONDON
LONDRA
LONDYN
LONG
LONI
LONNIE
LORA
LORAINE
LORALEI
LORALYE
LORAN
LORAND
LORCAN
LORD
LORDINA
LOREDANA

LOREEN
LORELAI
LORELEI
LORELIE
LORELL
LORELLA
LORELLE
LOREN
LORENA
LORENNA
LORENT
LORENZ
LORENZA
LORENZO
LORESA
LORETA
LORETTA
LORI
LORIANA
LORIANNE
LORIE
LORIEN
LORIK
LORIMER
LORIN
LORINA
LORINE
LORIS
LORISSA
LORNA
LORNA-JEAN
LORNE
LORRAINE
LORRELLE
LORREN
LORRENA
LORRETTA
LORRIE
LORYN
LOTANNA
LOTFI
LOTI
LOTTA
LOTTE
LOTTI
LOTTIE
LOTTIE-BELLE
LOTTIE-GRACE

LOTTIE-LEIGH	LOULIA	LUCA-JAMES
LOTTIE-LOU	LOULOU	LUCA-JAY
LOTTIE-LOUISE	LOURDES	LUCAH
LOTTIE-MAE	LOURENCO	LUCAIS
LOTTIE-MAI	LOURENS	LUCAN
LOTTIE-MARIE	LOUSHA	LUCAS
LOTTIE-MAY	LOVE	LUCAS-JACK
LOTTIE-RAE	LOVEDAY	LUCAS-JAMES
LOTTIE-ROSE	LOVELEEN	LUCAS-JAY
LOTTY	LOVELL	LUCAS-JOHN
LOTUS	LOVELLA	LUCAS-KAI
LOU	LOVELLE	LUCAS-LEE
LOU-ANNA	LOVELY	LUCAS-SCOTT
LOU-LOU	LOVINA	LUCCA
LOUANNA	LOVISA	LUCCAS
LOUANNE	LOWAN	LUCCIA
LOUAY	LOWE	LUCEA
LOUCA	LOWELL	LUCEE
LOUCAS	LOWEN	LUCEY
LOUEE	LOWENA	LUCHIA
LOUELLA	LOWENNA	LUCI
LOUEN	LOWIS	LUCI-JO
LOUEY	LOWRI	LUCIA
LOUGHLIN	LOWRIE	LUCIA-ROSE
LOUI	LOXIE	LUCIAN
LOUIE	LOXLEY	LUCIANA
LOUIE-GEORGE	LOXY	LUCIANNA
LOUIE-JAMES	LOYD	LUCIANNE
LOUIE-JAY	LOZA	LUCIANO
LOUIE-JOE	LU'AY	LUCIE
LOUIE-JOHN	LUA	LUCIE-ANN
LOUIS	LUAN	LUCIE-ANNE
LOUIS-JAMES	LUANA	LUCIE-JO
LOUISA	LUANNA	LUCIE-LOU
LOUISA-MAE	LUANNE	LUCIE-MAE
LOUISA-MAY	LUAY	LUCIE-MAI
LOUISA-ROSE	LUBAABAH	LUCIE-MAY
LOUISE	LUBABA	LUCIE-ROSE
LOUISHA	LUBABAH	LUCIEN
LOUISIANA	LUBELIHLE	LUCIENNA
LOUISIANNA	LUBNA	LUCIENNE
LOUIX	LUBNAA	LUCIFER
LOUIZA	LUBOMIR	LUCIJA
LOUJAIN	LUBOS	LUCILE
LOUKA	LUC	LUCILLA
LOUKAS	LUCA	LUCILLE
LOUKIA	LUCA-GABRIEL	LUCINA
LOULA	LUCA-GEORGE	LUCINDA

LUCINE
LUCIO
LUCION
LUCIOUS
LUCIUS
LUCJA
LUCJAN
LUCKY
LUCRETIA
LUCREZIA
LUCUS
LUCY
LUCY-
LUCY-ANN
LUCY-ANNA
LUCY-ANNE
LUCY-ELLEN
LUCY-JANE
LUCY-JAYNE
LUCY-JO
LUCY-LEIGH
LUCY-LOU
LUCY-LOUISE
LUCY-MAE
LUCY-MAI
LUCY-MARIE
LUCY-MAY
LUCY-RAE
LUCY-ROSE
LUCYANN
LUCYANNA
LUCYANNE
LUCYNA
LUDMILA
LUDO
LUDOVIC
LUDOVICA
LUDOVICO
LUDWIG
LUDWIK
LUELLA
LUEN
LUENA
LUEY
LUGHAN
LUI
LUIE
LUIGI

LUIS
LUISA
LUISE
LUIZ
LUIZA
LUIZE
LUJAIN
LUJAINE
LUJANE
LUJAYN
LUJZA
LUKA
LUKAH
LUKAS
LUKASH
LUKASZ
LUKE
LUKE-JAMES
LUKE-JUNIOR
LUKEN
LUKMAAN
LUKMAN
LUKNE
LUKRECIA
LUKRECIJA
LUKRECJA
LUKUS
LUL
LULA
LULA-BELLE
LULA-ROSE
LULABELLE
LULAH
LULIA
LULLAH
LULU
LULUA
LULYA
LULYANA
LUMEN
LUMI
LUNA
LUNA-BELLE
LUNA-MAE
LUNA-MAI
LUNA-MAY
LUNA-RAE
LUNA-ROSE

LUNAR
LUNASHA
LUNED
LUNNA
LUO
LUPE
LUQA
LUQMAAN
LUQMAN
LURA
LUSIA
LUSIANA
LUTFI
LUTFIYA
LUTFIYAH
LUTHANDO
LUTHER
LUUK
LUUL
LUV
LUWAM
LUX
LUXMI
LUYANDA
LUZ
LWANDLE
LWSI
LYA
LYAH
LYALL
LYAM
LYAN
LYANA
LYANNA
LYARA
LYAS
LYBA
LYBAH
LYCAN
LYCIA
LYDIA
LYDIA-GRACE
LYDIA-MAE
LYDIA-MAY
LYDIA-ROSE
LYDIE
LYDON
LYES

LYLA
LYLA-BELLE
LYLA-GRACE
LYLA-MAE
LYLA-MAI
LYLA-MAY
LYLA-RAE
LYLA-ROSE
LYLAH
LYLAH-ROSE
LYLE
LYLIA
LYLIE
LYN
LYNA
LYNCOLN
LYNCON
LYNDA
LYNDAN
LYNDEN
LYNDON
LYNDSAY
LYNDSEY
LYNETTE
LYNN
LYNNE
LYNNETTE
LYNSAY
LYNSEY
LYNTON
LYON
LYRA
LYRA-MAE
LYRA-MAY
LYRA-ROSE
LYRAH
LYRIC
LYSANDER
LYSETTE
LYSSA
LYSSIA
LYUBOV
LYVIA
LYZA

M

M
M'KAI
MA
MA'AZ
MAAB
MAAHI
MAAHIN
MAAHIR
MAAHIRA
MAAHIRAH
MAAHNOOR
MAAHUM
MAAIDA
MAAIKE
MAALI
MAALIK
MAALIKAH
MAAME
MAAN
MAANAS
MAANAV
MAANI
MAANSI
MAANVI
MAANYA
MAARIA
MAARIAH
MAARIYA
MAARIYAAH
MAARIYAH
MAARYA
MAAWA
MAAYA
MAAYAN
MAAZ
MAAZIN
MABEL
MABELLE
MABINTY
MABLE
MABLI
MABON
MAC
MACARA

MACARIO
MACAULAY
MACAULEE
MACAULEY
MACAULLAY
MACAULLEY
MACAULLY
MACAULY
MACAWLEY
MACAYLA
MACCAULEY
MACE
MACEE
MACEN
MACENZIE
MACEO
MACEY
MACEY-JANE
MACEY-JAYNE
MACEY-JO
MACEY-LEA
MACEY-LEE
MACEY-LEIGH
MACEY-LOU
MACEY-MAE
MACEY-MAY
MACEY-RAE
MACEY-ROSE
MACHAELA
MACHEDA
MACI
MACI-GRACE
MACI-JAI
MACI-LEA
MACI-LEIGH
MACI-MAE
MACI-MARIE
MACI-RAE
MACI-ROSE
MACIE
MACIE-ANN
MACIE-ANNE
MACIE-JANE
MACIE-JAY
MACIE-JO
MACIE-LEA
MACIE-LEE
MACIE-LEIGH

MACIE-LOU
MACIE-LOUISE
MACIE-MAE
MACIE-MAI
MACIE-MARIE
MACIE-MAY
MACIE-RAE
MACIE-ROSE
MACIEJ
MACIEK
MACK
MACKAI
MACKAYLA
MACKENNA
MACKENSEY
MACKENSIE
MACKENZI
MACKENZIE
MACKENZIE-LEE
MACKENZIE-LEIGH
MACKENZY
MACKINLEY
MACKLIN
MACKY
MACLAREN
MACORLEY
MACS
MACSEN
MACY
MACY-GRACE
MACY-JANE
MACY-JO
MACY-LEE
MACY-LEIGH
MACY-MAE
MACY-RAE
MACY-ROSE
MADALAINE
MADALEINE
MADALENA
MADALENE
MADALIN
MADALINA
MADALINE
MADALYN
MADALYNE
MADALYNN
MADALYNNE

MADAR	MADHIYA	MAELLE
MADARA	MADHVI	MAELLYS
MADDALENA	MADI	MAELONA
MADDALENE	MADIA	MAELY
MADDALYN	MADIAH	MAELYS
MADDELINE	MADIE	MAEMI
MADDEN	MADIHA	MAESHA
MADDI	MADIHAH	MAESIE
MADDIE	MADILYN	MAESON
MADDIE-LEIGH	MADINA	MAEVA
MADDIE-MAI	MADINAH	MAEVE
MADDIE-MAY	MADISEN	MAEYA
MADDIE-ROSE	MADISON	MAEZIE
MADDISEN	MADISON-GRACE	MAFALDA
MADDISON	MADISON-LEIGH	MAGALI
MADDISON-GRACE	MADISON-MAE	MAGAN
MADDISON-LEE	MADISON-MAY	MAGATHI
MADDISON-LEIGH	MADISON-ROSE	MAGDA
MADDISON-MAE	MADISSON	MAGDALEN
MADDISON-MAI	MADISYN	MAGDALENA
MADDISON-MAY	MADIYA	MAGDALENE
MADDISON-RAE	MADIYAH	MAGEN
MADDISON-ROSE	MADIYYAH	MAGENTA
MADDISSON	MADLEN	MAGGI
MADDISYN	MADLYN	MAGGIE
MADDIX	MADOC	MAGGIE-ANN
MADDOX	MADOG	MAGGIE-ANNE
MADDY	MADOKA	MAGGIE-JO
MADDYSON	MADONA	MAGGIE-MAE
MADEEHA	MADONNA	MAGGIE-MAI
MADEEHAH	MADOX	MAGGIE-MAY
MADEENAH	MADS	MAGGIE-ROSE
MADEHA	MADYAN	MAGI
MADELAINE	MADYSON	MAGNOLIA
MADELEINA	MAE	MAGNUS
MADELEINE	MAEA	MAGOR
MADELENA	MAEBEL	MAH
MADELENE	MAEBH	MAH-NOOR
MADELIEF	MAEBY	MAHA
MADELIENE	MAEDA	MAHAAN
MADELIN	MAEEN	MAHAD
MADELINE	MAEESHA	MAHADEV
MADELYN	MAEGAN	MAHADO
MADELYNE	MAEGHAN	MAHAK
MADELYNN	MAEL	MAHALA
MADHAV	MAELA	MAHALIA
MADHAVI	MAELEIGH	MAHAM
MADHIA	MAELIE	MAHAMAD

MAHAMARAKKALAGE
MAHAMED
MAHAMEDAMIN
MAHAMMAD
MAHAMMED
MAHAMOOD
MAHAMOUD
MAHAMUD
MAHAN
MAHANOOR
MAHATHI
MAHATHY
MAHAVEER
MAHAZ
MAHBEER
MAHBIR
MAHBOOB
MAHBUB
MAHBUBA
MAHBUBUL
MAHBUBUR
MAHD
MAHDEE
MAHDI
MAHDIA
MAHDIYA
MAHDIYAH
MAHDIYYA
MAHDIYYAH
MAHDY
MAHE
MAHEE
MAHEEMA
MAHEEN
MAHEER
MAHEERA
MAHEK
MAHEMA
MAHENOOR
MAHER
MAHERA
MAHESH
MAHFOOZ
MAHFUJ
MAHFUJUR
MAHFUZ
MAHFUZA
MAHFUZAH

MAHFUZUR
MAHI
MAHIA
MAHIB
MAHIBA
MAHIBAH
MAHID
MAHIDA
MAHIDUL
MAHIDUR
MAHIKA
MAHIM
MAHIMA
MAHIN
MAHINUR
MAHIR
MAHIRA
MAHIRAH
MAHIRUL
MAHISHA
MAHITH
MAHITHA
MAHIYA
MAHJABEEN
MAHJABIN
MAHLA
MAHLET
MAHLI
MAHLIA
MAHMOOD
MAHMOUD
MAHMUD
MAHMUDA
MAHMUDUL
MAHMUT
MAHNAZ
MAHNI
MAHNOOR
MAHNUR
MAHO
MAHOMED
MAHRA
MAHREEN
MAHREZ
MAHRIA
MAHRIN
MAHROSH
MAHRUKH

MAHRUS
MAHSA
MAHSAA
MAHTAB
MAHUM
MAHVEEN
MAHVESH
MAHVISH
MAHWISH
MAHZABIN
MAI
MAIA
MAIA-GRACE
MAIA-ROSE
MAIAH
MAICEE
MAICEY
MAICEY-LEIGH
MAICI
MAICIE
MAICIE-LEE
MAICIE-RAE
MAICY
MAIDA
MAIDAH
MAIDIE
MAIESHA
MAIGAN
MAIJA
MAIKA
MAIKLS
MAILA
MAILE
MAILEE
MAILEY
MAILI
MAILIE
MAILY
MAIMIE
MAIMOONA
MAIMOONAH
MAIMOUNA
MAIMUNA
MAIMUNAH
MAIR
MAIRA
MAIRAH
MAIRE

MAIREAD	MAISY-ANN	MAKAAY
MAIRI	MAISY-GRACE	MAKAEEL
MAIRIN	MAISY-JANE	MAKAELA
MAIRWEN	MAISY-JAYNE	MAKAI
MAIS	MAISY-LEIGH	MAKAIL
MAISA	MAISY-LOUISE	MAKAILA
MAISAH	MAISY-MAE	MAKAIO
MAISAM	MAISY-MAY	MAKALA
MAISARA	MAISY-RAE	MAKAN
MAISARAH	MAISY-ROSE	MAKANA
MAISE	MAITA	MAKANAKA
MAISEE	MAITE	MAKAR
MAISEY	MAITHAM	MAKARI
MAISEY-JANE	MAITHILI	MAKARIOS
MAISEY-LEIGH	MAITRI	MAKATENDEKA
MAISEY-RAE	MAIVISH	MAKAYLA
MAISEY-ROSE	MAIWAND	MAKDA
MAISHA	MAIWEN	MAKEBA
MAISHAH	MAIYA	MAKEDA
MAISI	MAIYAH	MAKEL
MAISIE	MAIZA	MAKENA
MAISIE-	MAIZAH	MAKENNA
MAISIE-ANN	MAIZE	MAKENZI
MAISIE-ANNE	MAIZEE	MAKENZIE
MAISIE-GRACE	MAIZEY	MAKENZY
MAISIE-JADE	MAIZI	MAKHAN
MAISIE-JAE	MAIZIE	MAKHI
MAISIE-JANE	MAIZIE-GRACE	MAKI
MAISIE-JAY	MAIZIE-LEIGH	MAKISHA
MAISIE-JAYNE	MAIZIE-MAE	MAKITA
MAISIE-JEAN	MAIZIE-ROSE	MAKKIYAH
MAISIE-JO	MAIZY	MAKO
MAISIE-LEA	MAJA	MAKOMBORERO
MAISIE-LEE	MAJD	MAKS
MAISIE-LEIGH	MAJED	MAKSIM
MAISIE-LOU	MAJEDA	MAKSIMILIAN
MAISIE-LOUISE	MAJEED	MAKSIMS
MAISIE-MAE	MAJELLA	MAKSYM
MAISIE-MAI	MAJENTA	MAKSYMILIAN
MAISIE-MARIE	MAJESTY	MAKYLA
MAISIE-MAY	MAJHARUL	MAL
MAISIE-RAE	MAJID	MALA
MAISIE-ROSE	MAJIDA	MALAAK
MAISIE-SUE	MAJIDAH	MALACHAI
MAISON	MAJKA	MALACHI
MAISON-LEE	MAJOR	MALACHIE
MAISSA	MAJUS	MALACHY
MAISY	MAK	MALACKI

MALAEKA
MALAIKA
MALAIKAH
MALAIKHA
MALAIQA
MALAK
MALAKAI
MALAKEY
MALAKHAI
MALAKHI
MALAKI
MALAKIA
MALAKIE
MALAKYE
MALALA
MALALAI
MALAN
MALANDRA
MALAYA
MALAYAH
MALAYEKA
MALAYKA
MALAYSIA
MALAZ
MALCOLM
MALCOM
MALEA
MALEAH
MALEEHA
MALEEHAH
MALEEK
MALEEKA
MALEEKAH
MALEHA
MALEIK
MALEIKA
MALEK
MALEKA
MALEN
MALENA
MALGORZATA
MALI
MALIA
MALIAH
MALIAKA
MALICA
MALICK
MALIE

MALIEK
MALIEKA
MALIHA
MALIHAH
MALIK
MALIKA
MALIKAH
MALIKAI
MALIKHA
MALIKI
MALIKYE
MALIN
MALINA
MALINI
MALIQ
MALIQUE
MALISA
MALISE
MALISHA
MALISSA
MALIYA
MALIYAH
MALIYKA
MALK
MALKA
MALKI
MALKIT
MALKY
MALLAK
MALLIE
MALLIKA
MALLK
MALLORY
MALLY
MALO
MALONE
MALOU
MALU
MALVIKA
MALVIN
MALVINA
MALWINA
MALYKA
MALYUN
MAM
MAMA
MAMADI
MAMADOU

MAMADU
MAME
MAMIE
MAMOON
MAMOONA
MAMOUDOU
MAMTA
MAMUN
MAMUNA
MAMUNUR
MAN
MANA
MANAAHIL
MANAAL
MANAHAL
MANAHEL
MANAHIL
MANAL
MANAN
MANAR
MANAS
MANASA
MANASI
MANASSE
MANASSEH
MANASVI
MANAT
MANAV
MANAVI
MANDANA
MANDEEP
MANDIP
MANDIPA
MANDISA
MANDY
MANEESHA
MANEET
MANEL
MANELLE
MANESH
MANESHA
MANFRED
MANH
MANHA
MANI
MANICHE
MANIKA
MANINDER

MANISH	MANTHAN	MARCIN
MANISHA	MANTRA	MARCIO
MANIT	MANU	MARCO
MANJINDER	MANUEL	MARCOS
MANJIT	MANUELA	MARCU
MANJOT	MANUELLA	MARCUS
MANKARAN	MANUS	MARCUS-LEE
MANKIRAN	MANVEEN	MARCY
MANKIRAT	MANVEER	MARD
MANLEEN	MANVI	MARDIN
MANMEET	MANVIK	MARDIYA
MANMOHAN	MANVINDER	MARDOCHEE
MANN	MANVIR	MAREA
MANNA	MANYA	MARED
MANNAN	MAPLE	MAREEHA
MANNAT	MAQADAS	MAREEN
MANNI	MAR	MAREENA
MANNIX	MARA	MAREK
MANNY	MARAH	MAREKS
MANOJ	MARAKI	MARELLA
MANOLO	MARAL	MAREN
MANOLYA	MARAM	MARENA
MANON	MARANATHA	MAREYA
MANOOR	MARAT	MARGARET
MANPREET	MARAYA	MARGARETA
MANPRIYA	MARAYAH	MARGARIDA
MANRAAJ	MARC	MARGARITA
MANRAJ	MARC-ANTHONY	MARGAUX
MANREET	MARCAS	MARGED
MANROOP	MARCEAU	MARGHERITA
MANSA	MARCEL	MARGITA
MANSEERAT	MARCELA	MARGO
MANSHA	MARCELI	MARGOT
MANSI	MARCELINA	MARGUERITA
MANSIMRAN	MARCELINE	MARGUERITE
MANSIRAT	MARCELINO	MARI
MANSON	MARCELL	MARI-ANNE
MANSOOR	MARCELLA	MARIA
MANSOR	MARCELLE	MARIA-LILY
MANSOUR	MARCELLO	MARIA-ROSE
MANSUKH	MARCELLUS	MARIAH
MANSUR	MARCELO	MARIAM
MANSURAH	MARCEY	MARIAMA
MANSUUR	MARCI	MARIAME
MANTAS	MARCIA	MARIAN
MANTASHA	MARCIANO	MARIANA
MANTE	MARCIE	MARIANNA
MANTEJ	MARCIE-MAE	MARIANNE

MARIATOU	MARIYAH	MARLIE-MAE
MARIBEL	MARIYAM	MARLIN
MARICA	MARIYAMBIBI	MARLO
MARIE	MARIYUM	MARLOE
MARIE-ANNE	MARIYYAH	MARLON
MARIE-CLAIRE	MARIZA	MARLOW
MARIE-LOUISE	MARJAAN	MARLOWE
MARIEKE	MARJAN	MARLY
MARIEL	MARJANA	MARMADUKE
MARIELA	MARJIA	MARNEE
MARIELLA	MARJORIE	MARNEY
MARIELLE	MARK	MARNI
MARIEM	MARK-	MARNI-ROSE
MARIEME	MARK-JUNIOR	MARNIA
MARIESHA	MARKAS	MARNIE
MARIETTA	MARKEL	MARNIE-GRACE
MARIETTE	MARKELL	MARNIE-LEIGH
MARIGOLD	MARKETA	MARNIE-MAE
MARIHA	MARKIYAN	MARNIE-MAI
MARIHAH	MARKO	MARNIE-MAY
MARIJA	MARKOS	MARNIE-RAE
MARIJUS	MARKS	MARNIE-ROSE
MARIKA	MARKUS	MARNY
MARIKO	MARKUSS	MARO
MARILENA	MARKY	MAROOF
MARILIA	MARLA	MAROS
MARILLA	MARLEA	MAROUANE
MARILYN	MARLEE	MARQUES
MARIN	MARLEE-GRACE	MARQUEZ
MARINA	MARLEE-MAE	MARQUIS
MARINE	MARLEEN	MARQUISE
MARINO	MARLEI	MARRIA
MARIO	MARLEIGH	MARRIAM
MARIOM	MARLEN	MARRISA
MARION	MARLENA	MARRISSA
MARIOS	MARLENE	MARRIUM
MARIS	MARLEY	MARRIYAH
MARISA	MARLEY-GRACE	MARSDEN
MARISHA	MARLEY-JAI	MARSEL
MARISKA	MARLEY-JAMES	MARSELA
MARISOL	MARLEY-JAY	MARSHA
MARISSA	MARLEY-JOE	MARSHAL
MARITA	MARLEY-LEE	MARSHALL
MARIUM	MARLEY-MAE	MARSHALL-LEE
MARIUS	MARLEY-RAE	MARTA
MARIUSZ	MARLEY-ROSE	MARTEL
MARIYA	MARLI	MARTELL
MARIYAAH	MARLIE	MARTHA

MARTHA-GRACE	MARY-JANE	MASON
MARTHA-LILY	MARY-JAYNE	MASON-JAMES
MARTHA-MAE	MARY-JEAN	MASON-JAY
MARTHA-MAI	MARY-JO	MASON-JOHN
MARTHA-MAY	MARY-KATE	MASON-LEE
MARTHA-ROSE	MARY-LOU	MASON-LEIGH
MARTI	MARY-LOUISE	MASON-RILEY
MARTIA	MARY-ROSE	MASON-THOMAS
MARTIAL	MARYA	MASOOD
MARTIJN	MARYAH	MASOOM
MARTIKA	MARYAM	MASOOMA
MARTIM	MARYAMA	MASOOMAH
MARTIN	MARYAN	MASOUD
MARTINA	MARYANN	MASROOR
MARTINAS	MARYANNA	MASRUR
MARTINE	MARYANNE	MASSA
MARTINIQUE	MARYBETH	MASSI
MARTINO	MARYELLEN	MASSIMILIANO
MARTINS	MARYEM	MASSIMO
MARTON	MARYIA	MASSON
MARTY	MARYIAM	MASUD
MARTYN	MARYIM	MASUDUR
MARTYNA	MARYJANE	MASUM
MARTYNAS	MARYKATE	MASUMA
MARUF	MARYLA	MASUMAH
MARUKH	MARYLOU	MASUUD
MARVA	MARYLYN	MAT
MARVEL	MARYO	MATAEO
MARVELLOUS	MARYROSE	MATAI
MARVELOUS	MARYSIA	MATAIO
MARVI	MARYUM	MATAN
MARVIN	MARZANA	MATAS
MARVYN	MARZIA	MATAYA
MARWA	MARZUQ	MATE
MARWAAN	MASA	MATEA
MARWAH	MASAL	MATEEN
MARWAN	MASE	MATEI
MARWO	MASEEH	MATEJ
MARWOOD	MASEN	MATEJA
MARY	MASEY	MATEJUS
MARY-	MASHA	MATEL
MARY-ANN	MASHAL	MATEN
MARY-ANNA	MASHIYAT	MATEO
MARY-ANNE	MASHUD	MATEOS
MARY-BETH	MASIE	MATEUS
MARY-ELIZABETH	MASIEY	MATEUSZ
MARY-ELLEN	MASIH	MATEY
MARY-GRACE	MASIMBA	MATH

MATHEA
MATHEO
MATHEUS
MATHEW
MATHEWS
MATHIAS
MATHIEU
MATHILDA
MATHILDE
MATHIS
MATHUMITHA
MATHURA
MATHUSAN
MATHUSHA
MATHUSHAN
MATHYS
MATI
MATIA
MATIAS
MATIDA
MATIFADZA
MATILDA
MATILDA-MAE
MATILDA-MAY
MATILDA-RAE
MATILDA-ROSE
MATILDE
MATIN
MATIS
MATISS
MATISSE
MATS
MATT
MATTEA
MATTEO
MATTEUS
MATTHAUS
MATTHEO
MATTHEUS
MATTHEW
MATTHEW-JAMES
MATTHEWS
MATTHIAS
MATTHIEU
MATTHIJS
MATTHIS
MATTHYS
MATTI
MATTIA
MATTIAS
MATTIE
MATTILDA
MATTIS
MATTY
MATUS
MATVEI
MATVEJ
MATVEY
MATVIY
MATYAS
MATYLDA
MATYS
MAUD
MAUDE
MAULI
MAULIK
MAURA
MAUREEN
MAURICE
MAURICIO
MAURISIO
MAURITS
MAURIZIO
MAURO
MAURYCY
MAVEN
MAVERICK
MAVI
MAVIS
MAVISH
MAVISHA
MAVLEEN
MAVRICK
MAWA
MAWADA
MAWADAH
MAWADDA
MAWADDAH
MAWAHIB
MAWGAN
MAWIYAH
MAX
MAXAMILIAN
MAXAMILLIAN
MAXAMILLION
MAXEN
MAXENCE
MAXFIELD
MAXI
MAXIE
MAXIM
MAXIMA
MAXIME
MAXIMILIAN
MAXIMILIANO
MAXIMILIEN
MAXIMILLIAN
MAXIMILLION
MAXIMO
MAXIMOS
MAXIMUS
MAXINE
MAXMILIAN
MAXON
MAXSON
MAXTON
MAXWEL
MAXWELL
MAXX
MAXXIE
MAXYMILIAN
MAXYMILLIAN
MAY
MAYA
MAYA-ROSE
MAYAH
MAYAMEEN
MAYAMIKO
MAYAN
MAYANA
MAYANK
MAYAR
MAYARA
MAYAS
MAYBEL
MAYBELLE
MAYCE
MAYCEE
MAYCI
MAYCIE
MAYCIE-LEIGH
MAYDA
MAYE
MAYEDA

MAYER	MAZIE	MEDEEA
MAYESHA	MAZIE-LEIGH	MEDEEHA
MAYGAN	MAZIN	MEDEINA
MAYIA	MAZLUM	MEDHA
MAYISHA	MAZVITA	MEDHANSH
MAYLA	MAZY	MEDI
MAYLE	MBALENHLE	MEDINA
MAYLEE	MC	MEDINAH
MAYLEIGH	MCALLISTER	MEDINE
MAYLI	MCAULEY	MEDWYN
MAYLIE	MCCARTNEY	MEEGAN
MAYLIN	MCCAULAY	MEEKA
MAYLY	MCCAULEY	MEEKAH
MAYMOONA	MCCAULLEY	MEEKAL
MAYMOONAH	MCCAWLEY	MEELA
MAYMUNA	MCCORLEY	MEELAH
MAYMUNAH	MCCOY	MEENA
MAYNARD	MCKAI	MEENAKSHI
MAYON	MCKAYLA	MEER
MAYOWA	MCKENNA	MEERA
MAYRA	MCKENZEE	MEERAB
MAYS	MCKENZI	MEERUB
MAYSA	MCKENZIE	MEESAM
MAYSAA	MCKENZIE-JAMES	MEESHA
MAYSAM	MCKENZIE-JAY	MEESUM
MAYSARAH	MCKENZIE-JOHN	MEET
MAYSHA	MCKENZIE-LEE	MEEYA
MAYSIE	MCKENZIE-LEIGH	MEG
MAYSON	MCKENZY	MEGAN
MAYSOON	MCKINLEY	MEGAN-ANNE
MAYSSA	MCKYE	MEGAN-GRACE
MAYSUN	MCKYLA	MEGAN-LEIGH
MAYSUUN	MCLAREN	MEGAN-LOUISE
MAYTAL	MD	MEGAN-MARIE
MAYU	MD.	MEGAN-ROSE
MAYUKHA	MDUDUZI	MEGANE
MAYUMI	MEA	MEGANN
MAYUR	MEABH	MEGANNE
MAYURI	MEADHBH	MEGEN
MAYYA	MEADOW	MEGGAN
MAYZEE	MEAGAN	MEGGIE
MAYZI	MEAGHAN	MEGH
MAYZIE	MEAH	MEGHA
MAZEDA	MEARA	MEGHAN
MAZEN	MEASHA	MEGHAN-ROSE
MAZEY	MEAVE	MEGHANA
MAZHAR	MECHEL	MEGHANE
MAZHARUL	MEDA	MEGHANN

MEGHNA
MEGI
MEGIJA
MEGUMI
MEGYN
MEHA
MEHAK
MEHAR
MEHBOOB
MEHDI
MEHEK
MEHER
MEHGAN
MEHJABEEN
MEHJABIN
MEHMA
MEHMED
MEHMET
MEHMOONA
MEHNAAZ
MEHNAZ
MEHNOOR
MEHR
MEHRAAB
MEHRAAN
MEHRAB
MEHRAJ
MEHRAN
MEHRAZ
MEHREEN
MEHRIN
MEHRISH
MEHRUN
MEHRUNNISA
MEHTAAB
MEHTAB
MEHUL
MEHVISH
MEHWISH
MEHZABIN
MEI
MEI-LING
MEIA
MEIDA
MEIKA
MEIKE
MEILA
MEILANI
MEILECH
MEILI
MEILIR
MEILYR
MEINIR
MEIR
MEIRA
MEIRION
MEISHA
MEITAL
MEJA
MEKA
MEKAAL
MEKAI
MEKAIL
MEKAYLA
MEKEDA
MEKENZIE
MEKHAI
MEKHI
MEKLIT
MEL
MELA
MELAD
MELAHER
MELAINA
MELAINE
MELAK
MELANI
MELANIA
MELANIE
MELANIJA
MELANY
MELAT
MELCHIZEDEK
MELDA
MELEAH
MELEK
MELENA
MELERI
MELIA
MELIAH
MELIH
MELIHA
MELIK
MELIKA
MELIKE
MELINA
MELINDA
MELIS
MELISA
MELISE
MELISHA
MELISSA
MELITA
MELIYAH
MELIZ
MELLIEHA
MELLINA
MELLISA
MELLISSA
MELODEE
MELODI
MELODIE
MELODY
MELODY-MAY
MELODY-ROSE
MELTEM
MELVIN
MELVINA
MELVYN
MELWIN
MELYSSA
MEMET
MEMOONA
MEMPHIS
MEMUNA
MENA
MENAAL
MENACHEM
MENAHIL
MENAL
MENASHE
MENDEL
MENDY
MENELIK
MENG
MENISHA
MENNA
MERA
MERAB
MERAJ
MERAL
MERAN
MERCADES
MERCEDES

MERCEDEZ
MERCEDIE
MERCER
MERCI
MERCIA
MERCIE
MERCY
MERDAN
MERDI
MEREDITH
MEREDYDD
MEREDYTH
MEREL
MERGIM
MERI
MERIAM
MERIC
MERIDA
MERIDITH
MERIEL
MERIEM
MERILIN
MERILYN
MERIN
MERINA
MERIS
MERISSA
MERITA
MERITXELL
MERIYAM
MERLE
MERLIN
MERLYN
MERNA
MERON
MERREN
MERRICK
MERRIE
MERRILEES
MERRILL
MERRIN
MERRISSA
MERRY
MERRYN
MERSON
MERT
MERTCAN
MERVE

MERVEILLE
MERVIN
MERVYN
MERYAM
MERYEM
MERYL
MERYN
MESHA
MESHACH
MESHAQ
MESHILEM
MESHULEM
MESK
MESSI
MESSIAH
MESUM
META
METE
METEHAN
METHEMBE
METIN
METODI
METTE
MEURIG
MEVISH
MEYA
MEYAH
MEYER
MHAIRI
MHARI
MI
MIA
MIA-
MIA-ANN
MIA-ANNE
MIA-BELLA
MIA-BROOKE
MIA-FAITH
MIA-GRACE
MIA-JADE
MIA-JANE
MIA-JASMINE
MIA-JAY
MIA-JAYNE
MIA-JO
MIA-JOAN
MIA-LEIGH
MIA-LILLY

MIA-LILY
MIA-LOUISE
MIA-MAE
MIA-MAI
MIA-MARIE
MIA-MAY
MIA-NICOLE
MIA-PAIGE
MIA-RAE
MIA-RENEE
MIA-ROSE
MIA-SKYE
MIAA
MIABELLA
MIAH
MIAH-GRACE
MIAH-ROSE
MIAMI
MIAN
MIAR
MIAROSE
MIAYA
MICA
MICAEL
MICAELA
MICAH
MICAIAH
MICAYLA
MICHA
MICHAEL
MICHAEL-JAMES
MICHAEL-JOHN
MICHAEL-JUNIOR
MICHAEL-LEE
MICHAELA
MICHAELA-ROSE
MICHAELLA
MICHAI
MICHAIL
MICHAL
MICHALA
MICHALINA
MICHALIS
MICHEAL
MICHEALA
MICHEE
MICHEL
MICHELA

MICHELANGELO
MICHELE
MICHELLA
MICHELLE
MICHIEL
MICHLE
MICHOEL
MICIA
MICIAH
MICK
MICKAEL
MICKAELA
MICKAYLA
MICKEL
MICKELA
MICKEY
MICKI
MICKIE
MICKY
MICKYLE
MIDAS
MIDHUN
MIDORI
MIEKA
MIEKE
MIEL
MIELA
MIESHA
MIESZKO
MIGEL
MIGENA
MIGLE
MIGUEL
MIHAEL
MIHAELA
MIHAI
MIHAIL
MIHAILO
MIHAILS
MIHAJLO
MIHALY
MIHELI
MIHIKA
MIHIN
MIHIR
MIHNEA
MIHRAN
MIHRIBAN

MIIA
MIJA
MIJANUR
MIKA
MIKA'EEL
MIKA'IL
MIKAAL
MIKAEEL
MIKAEL
MIKAELA
MIKAELLA
MIKAH
MIKAI
MIKAIL
MIKAILA
MIKAL
MIKALA
MIKALAH
MIKAYA
MIKAYEEL
MIKAYELA
MIKAYLA
MIKAYLA-ROSE
MIKAYLAH
MIKE
MIKEAL
MIKEALA
MIKEE
MIKEL
MIKELA
MIKESH
MIKEY
MIKHAEEL
MIKHAEL
MIKHAELA
MIKHAIL
MIKHEL
MIKHELA
MIKHIL
MIKI
MIKIE
MIKILA
MIKKA
MIKKEL
MIKKI
MIKKO
MIKLOS
MIKO

MIKOLAJ
MIKS
MIKU
MIKYLA
MIKYLE
MILA
MILA-GRACE
MILA-MAE
MILA-RAE
MILA-ROSE
MILAD
MILADA
MILAGROS
MILAH
MILAN
MILANA
MILANAS
MILAND
MILANI
MILANIA
MILANNA
MILANO
MILCAH
MILDA
MILDRED
MILEENA
MILEIGH
MILEJA
MILEN
MILENA
MILES
MILETA
MILEY
MILEY-GRACE
MILEY-JO
MILEY-LOUISE
MILEY-MAE
MILEY-MAI
MILEY-MAY
MILEY-RAE
MILEY-ROSE
MILI
MILIA
MILIANA
MILICA
MILIKA
MILIND
MILISSA

MILITA	MILLY-MAY	MIQDAD
MILKA	MILLY-ROSE	MIQUEL
MILLA	MILO	MIR
MILLAN	MILOS	MIRA
MILLAR	MILOSZ	MIRAAL
MILLE	MILOU	MIRAB
MILLEE	MILTON	MIRABEL
MILLEN	MILUN	MIRABELLA
MILLENA	MIMI	MIRABELLE
MILLER	MIMOSA	MIRAC
MILLEY	MIN	MIRACLE
MILLI	MINA	MIRAH
MILLI-ANN	MINAAHIL	MIRAI
MILLIA	MINAAL	MIRAIN
MILLIANA	MINAH	MIRAJ
MILLICENT	MINAHAL	MIRAL
MILLIE	MINAHIL	MIRAN
MILLIE-	MINAL	MIRANDA
MILLIE-ANN	MINAMI	MIRAY
MILLIE-ANNE	MINDAUGAS	MIRAYA
MILLIE-AVA	MINDY	MIRAZ
MILLIE-BETH	MINE	MIRCEA
MILLIE-GRACE	MINERVA	MIREIA
MILLIE-JADE	MINESH	MIREILLE
MILLIE-JANE	MINETTE	MIREL
MILLIE-JAY	MING	MIRELA
MILLIE-JAYNE	MINH	MIRELLA
MILLIE-JO	MINHA	MIREN
MILLIE-KATE	MINHAJ	MIREYA
MILLIE-LEE	MINHAJUL	MIRHA
MILLIE-LEIGH	MINHAL	MIRI
MILLIE-LOUISE	MINHAZ	MIRIAM
MILLIE-MAE	MINHAZUL	MIRIAN
MILLIE-MAI	MINI	MIRIELLE
MILLIE-MARIE	MINKA	MIRKO
MILLIE-MAY	MINKE	MIRNA
MILLIE-RAE	MINNA	MIRO
MILLIE-ROSE	MINNAH	MIRON
MILLIE-SUE	MINNI	MIROSLAV
MILLIEMAE	MINNIE	MIROSLAVA
MILLIGAN	MINNIE-MAE	MIRREN
MILLISA	MINNIE-RAE	MIRRI
MILLISSA	MINNIE-ROSE	MIRUNA
MILLY	MINNY	MIRWAIS
MILLY-ANN	MINSA	MIRYAM
MILLY-ANNE	MINUKI	MIRZA
MILLY-MAE	MINULI	MIRZAN
MILLY-MARIE	MIO	MISA

MISAKI	MITZI	MOFIYINFOLUWA
MISBA	MITZIE	MOFOPEFOLUWA
MISBAAH	MITZY	MOHAB
MISBAH	MIU	MOHAD
MISCHA	MIVAAN	MOHAK
MISEK	MIYA	MOHAMAD
MISHA	MIYAH	MOHAMED
MISHAAL	MIYAH-ROSE	MOHAMED-AMIN
MISHAEL	MIYANA	MOHAMEDAMIIN
MISHAL	MIYLA	MOHAMEDAMIN
MISHALL	MIYU	MOHAMMAD
MISHAN	MIYUKI	MOHAMMAD-ALI
MISHEEL	MIZAN	MOHAMMAD-AYAAN
MISHEL	MIZANUR	MOHAMMAD-HASSAN
MISHIKA	MIZGIN	MOHAMMAD-IBRAHIM
MISHKA	MIZUKI	MOHAMMAD-
MISHKAT	MJ	MUSTAFA
MISK	MKENZIE	MOHAMMAD-UMAR
MISKI	MLAK	MOHAMMAD-YUSUF
MISRI	MMESOMACHUKWU	MOHAMMED
MISSI	MO	MOHAMMED-
MISSIE	MO'NIQUE	MOHAMMED-ADAM
MISSY	MOAAD	MOHAMMED-ALI
MISTI	MOAAZ	MOHAMMED-ARMAAN
MISTY	MOAD	MOHAMMED-AYAAN
MISZEL	MOANA	MOHAMMED-DEEN
MITALI	MOAYAD	MOHAMMED-FARHAN
MITCH	MOAZ	MOHAMMED-HAMZA
MITCHAL	MOAZZAM	MOHAMMED-HASSAN
MITCHALL	MOBARAK	MOHAMMED-IBRAHIM
MITCHEL	MOBASHER	MOHAMMED-ISA
MITCHELL	MOBEEN	MOHAMMED-MUSA
MITCHELL-LEE	MOBEENA	MOHAMMED-MUSTAFA
MITCHUM	MOBIN	MOHAMMED-RAYYAN
MITEN	MOBINA	MOHAMMED-YAHYA
MITESH	MOBOLAJI	MOHAMMED-YUSUF
MITHIL	MODASER	MOHAMMED-
MITHRA	MODESIRE	ZAKARIYA
MITHRAN	MODESIREOLUWA	MOHAMMEDALI
MITHUN	MODOU	MOHAMMMED
MITHUSA	MODUPE	MOHAMMOD
MITHUSH	MOE	MOHAMMUD
MITHUSHA	MOEED	MOHAMOD
MITHUSHAN	MOEEN	MOHAMOUD
MITKO	MOEEZ	MOHAMUD
MITRA	MOESHA	MOHAN
MITUL	MOEZ	MOHANAD
MITZEE	MOFEOLUWA	MOHANED

MOHANNAD
MOHANNED
MOHBEEN
MOHD
MOHEED
MOHEEN
MOHEEZ
MOHEMA
MOHHAMED
MOHIB
MOHIBULLAH
MOHIBUR
MOHID
MOHIMA
MOHIN
MOHINI
MOHIT
MOHIUDDIN
MOHMED
MOHMMAD
MOHMMED
MOHNISH
MOHOMMED
MOHSAN
MOHSEN
MOHSIN
MOHSINA
MOHUMMED
MOI
MOIA
MOIN
MOINUDDIN
MOIRA
MOISE
MOISES
MOISHE
MOISHI
MOISHY
MOIZ
MOJOLAOLUWA
MOJTABA
MOKSH
MOKSHA
MOLI
MOLIK
MOLLEE
MOLLEY
MOLLI

MOLLIE
MOLLIE-
MOLLIE-ANN
MOLLIE-ANNE
MOLLIE-JANE
MOLLIE-JO
MOLLIE-LOUISE
MOLLIE-MAE
MOLLIE-MAI
MOLLIE-MAY
MOLLIE-RAE
MOLLIE-ROSE
MOLLY
MOLLY-
MOLLY-ANN
MOLLY-ANNE
MOLLY-GRACE
MOLLY-JANE
MOLLY-JO
MOLLY-LOUISE
MOLLY-MAE
MOLLY-MAI
MOLLY-MAY
MOLLY-RAE
MOLLY-ROSE
MOLLYANN
MOLLYANNE
MOLLYMAY
MOMAL
MOMEN
MOMENA
MOMIN
MOMINA
MOMINAH
MOMNA
MOMNAH
MOMO
MOMODOU
MOMOKA
MOMOKO
MOMOREOLUWA
MONA
MONAE
MONAI
MONALISA
MONAY
MONCEF
MONEEB

MONEEBA
MONEER
MONET
MONIA
MONIBA
MONICA
MONIFA
MONIFAH
MONIKA
MONIQUE
MONIR
MONIRA
MONISHA
MONISOLA
MONJUR
MONNAY
MONROE
MONTA
MONTAGU
MONTAGUE
MONTAHA
MONTANA
MONTANNA
MONTE
MONTEL
MONTELL
MONTELLE
MONTGOMERY
MONTI
MONTY
MOONISAH
MOOSA
MORAD
MORAG
MORAYO
MORAYOOLUWA
MORDCHE
MORDECAI
MORDECHAI
MORDECHI
MORENA
MORENIKE
MORGAN
MORGAN-
MORGAN-JAMES
MORGAN-LEE
MORGAN-LEIGH
MORGANA

MORGANE	MOSTYN	MUAZ
MORGANN	MOTIEJUS	MUAZZAM
MORGANNA	MOTTEL	MUBAARAK
MORGANNE	MOTTI	MUBARAK
MORGEN	MOTTY	MUBARAQ
MORGHAN	MOTUNRAYO	MUBAREK
MORGON	MOUAD	MUBARIK
MORIAH	MOUHAMADOU	MUBASHAR
MORIAM	MOUHAMED	MUBASHER
MORIOM	MOUHAMMED	MUBASHIR
MORIREOLUWA	MOUMIN	MUBASHSHIR
MORITZ	MOUNA	MUBASHSHIRAH
MORIUM	MOUNIR	MUBEEN
MORLEY	MOUNIRA	MUBIN
MORNA	MOURAD	MUDASER
MORNE	MOUSA	MUDASIR
MOROCCO	MOUSHUMI	MUDASSAR
MOROLAKE	MOUSSA	MUDASSIR
MORRIE	MOUSTAFA	MUDATHIR
MORRIGAN	MOUSTAPHA	MUDIWA
MORRIS	MOYA	MUEED
MORRISON	MOYINOLUWA	MUEEN
MORSAL	MOYNUL	MUEEZ
MORTAZA	MOYOSORE	MUFADDAL
MORTEN	MOYOSOREOLUWA	MUFARO
MORTIMER	MOZA	MUFAROWASHE
MORTON	MOZAN	MUHAB
MORUS	MOZES	MUHAIMIN
MORVEN	MTHABISI	MUHAMAD
MORVERN	MU'AAD	MUHAMADU
MORVYN	MU'AADH	MUHAMED
MORWENNA	MU'AAZ	MUHAMET
MOSA	MU'ADH	MUHAMMAD
MOSAB	MU'AWIYAH	MUHAMMAD-
MOSAMMAD	MU'MINAH	MUHAMMAD-ABDULLAH
MOSAMMAT	MUAAD	MUHAMMAD-ADAM
MOSAMMATH	MUAADH	MUHAMMAD-ALI
MOSAN	MUAAWIYAH	MUHAMMAD-AYAAN
MOSES	MUAAZ	MUHAMMAD-BILAL
MOSEY	MUAD	MUHAMMAD-DEEN
MOSHE	MUADH	MUHAMMAD-EESA
MOSHIN	MUAMMAR	MUHAMMAD-HAMZA
MOSIAH	MUATH	MUHAMMAD-HASHIM
MOSKA	MUAWIYAH	MUHAMMAD-HASSAAN
MOSOPEFOLUWA	MUAWWIZ	MUHAMMAD-HASSAN
MOSS	MUAYAD	MUHAMMAD-HUSSAIN
MOSSAMMAD	MUAYID	
MOSTAFA	MUAYYAD	

MUHAMMAD-IBRAHEEM
MUHAMMAD-IBRAHIM
MUHAMMAD-ISA
MUHAMMAD-ISMAEEL
MUHAMMAD-ISMAIL
MUHAMMAD-KAIF
MUHAMMAD-MUSA
MUHAMMAD-MUSTAFA
MUHAMMAD-RAYAN
MUHAMMAD-RAYYAN
MUHAMMAD-UMAR
MUHAMMAD-UZAIR
MUHAMMAD-YAHYA
MUHAMMAD-YOUSUF
MUHAMMAD-YUSUF
MUHAMMAD-ZAKARIYA
MUHAMMAD-ZAKARIYYA
MUHAMMAD-ZAYN
MUHAMMADALI
MUHAMMED
MUHAMMED-ALI
MUHAMMED-AYAAN
MUHAMMED-IBRAHIM
MUHAMMED-MUSA
MUHAMMET
MUHAMMOD
MUHAMMUD
MUHANAD
MUHANNAD
MUHAYMIN
MUHIB
MUHIBB
MUHIBUR
MUHMMAD
MUHSIN
MUHSINA
MUHSINAH
MUHTASIM
MUHUMMAD
MUHUMMED
MUID
MUIREANN
MUIZ
MUIZZ
MUIZZA

MUJAAHID
MUJAHID
MUJEEB
MUJIB
MUJIBUR
MUJTABA
MUKADAS
MUKARRAM
MUKESH
MUKHLISAH
MUKHTAR
MUKTAR
MUKTI
MUKUL
MUKUND
MULKI
MUMIN
MUMINA
MUMINAH
MUMTAHINA
MUMTAS
MUMTAZ
MUN
MUNA
MUNACHI
MUNACHIMSO
MUNACHISO
MUNASAR
MUNASHE
MUNAWAR
MUNAZZA
MUNDHIR
MUNEEB
MUNEEBA
MUNEEBAH
MUNEEF
MUNEEFA
MUNEER
MUNEERA
MUNEERAH
MUNEET
MUNEEZA
MUNESU
MUNEZA
MUNGO
MUNIB
MUNIBA
MUNIBAH

MUNIIRA
MUNIR
MUNIRA
MUNIRAH
MUNIRAT
MUNISA
MUNISAH
MUNRAJ
MUNRO
MUNSIF
MUNTAHA
MUNTASIR
MUNTAZ
MUNTAZIR
MUNYARADZI
MUQADAAS
MUQADAS
MUQADDAS
MUQEET
MUQTADIR
MURAAD
MURAD
MURAT
MURDO
MURDOCH
MURIAM
MURIEL
MURIUM
MURPHY
MURRAY
MURREN
MURRIN
MURRON
MURSAL
MURSALEEN
MURSHED
MURTADHA
MURTAZA
MUS'AB
MUSA
MUSAA
MUSAAB
MUSAB
MUSADDIQ
MUSAH
MUSAID
MUSAMMAD
MUSAMMAT

MUSAMMATH	MUZAMIL	MYLEA
MUSAMMED	MUZAMMIL	MYLEE
MUSAMMOD	MUZNA	MYLEE-MAE
MUSAMMOTH	MUZNAH	MYLEEN
MUSAWER	MUZZAMMIL	MYLEENE
MUSAWWIR	MY	MYLEI
MUSCAB	MYA	MYLEIGH
MUSE	MYA-GRACE	MYLENE
MUSEERAH	MYA-JANE	MYLES
MUSFIRAH	MYA-LEIGH	MYLEY
MUSHARRAF	MYA-LOUISE	MYLI
MUSHTABA	MYA-MAE	MYLIE
MUSHTAQ	MYA-MAI	MYLIE-MAI
MUSKA	MYA-MARIE	MYLIE-RAE
MUSKAAN	MYA-MAY	MYLO
MUSKAN	MYA-RAE	MYRA
MUSKHAN	MYA-ROSE	MYRAH
MUSLIM	MYAH	MYRAN
MUSLIMA	MYAH-GRACE	MYREEN
MUSLIMAH	MYAH-ROSE	MYRIAM
MUSSA	MYAN	MYRNA
MUSSAB	MYANNA	MYRON
MUSSAMAT	MYAR	MYRTLE
MUSSAMMAD	MYCAH	MYRTO
MUSSAMMAT	MYEESHA	MYSHA
MUSSAMMED	MYEISHA	MYTCHEL
MUSSE	MYER	
MUSTAF	MYESHA	
MUSTAFA	MYFANWY	
MUSTAFAA	MYFI	
MUSTAFAH	MYIA	
MUSTAFE	MYIAH	
MUSTAFIZUR	MYIESHA	
MUSTAKIM	MYKA	
MUSTANSIR	MYKAH	
MUSTAPHA	MYKAL	
MUSTAQEEM	MYKEL	
MUSTAQIM	MYKIE	
MUSTHAFA	MYKOLA	
MUSU	MYKOLAS	
MUTASIM	MYLA	
MUTMAINNAH	MYLA-MAE	
MUTSA	MYLA-MAY	
MUTSAWASHE	MYLA-RAE	
MUZAINA	MYLA-ROSE	
MUZAKIR	MYLAH	
MUZAKKIR	MYLAH-ROSE	
MUZAMEL	MYLAN	

N

NA
NA'EEMAH
NA'IL
NA'ILAH
NA'IMA
NAA
NAA'IL
NAADIA
NAADIR
NAADIYA
NAADIYAH
NAADRAH
NAAEL
NAAIL
NAAILA
NAAILAH
NAAIRAH
NAAMA
NAANA
NAAVYA
NAAYAAB
NAAYEL
NAAZISH
NABA
NABAA
NABEEHA
NABEEL
NABEELA
NABEELAH
NABEHA
NABHAAN
NABHAN
NABIA
NABIEL
NABIHA
NABIHAH
NABIIL
NABIL
NABILA
NABILAH
NABIYA
NACERA
NACHMAN
NACHMEN

NACIMO
NADA
NADAH
NADAL
NADAV
NADEEM
NADEEN
NADEERA
NADEJDA
NADENE
NADER
NADERA
NADEZHDA
NADHIA
NADHIR
NADIA
NADIAH
NADIIR
NADIM
NADIMA
NADIN
NADINA
NADINE
NADIR
NADIRA
NADIRAH
NADISHA
NADIYA
NADIYAH
NADJA
NADRA
NADYA
NADYNE
NAEEM
NAEEMA
NAEEMAH
NAEL
NAEMA
NAETOCHUKWU
NAEVE
NAEVIA
NAFEES
NAFEESA
NAFEESAH
NAFEEZA
NAFESA
NAFIA
NAFIS

NAFISA
NAFISAH
NAFISHA
NAFIZA
NAFTALI
NAFTOLI
NAFTULI
NAGA
NAGAD
NAGEENA
NAGINA
NAGLIS
NAGMA
NAHAL
NAHEDA
NAHEED
NAHEEDA
NAHEEDAH
NAHEEM
NAHEL
NAHEMA
NAHI
NAHIA
NAHIAN
NAHID
NAHIDA
NAHIDAH
NAHIDUL
NAHIL
NAHIM
NAHIMA
NAHIN
NAHIYA
NAHIYAN
NAHLA
NAHOM
NAHOME
NAHSHON
NAHUM
NAHYAAN
NAHYAN
NAIA
NAIARA
NAIDA
NAIEL
NAIF
NAIHA
NAILA

NAILAH	NAKEISHA	NANCY
NAIM	NAKIA	NANCY-JANE
NAIMA	NAKISHA	NANCY-LEE
NAIMAH	NAKITA	NANCY-LEIGH
NAIMAT	NAKIYAH	NANCY-LOU
NAIMH	NAKSH	NANCY-MAE
NAIMUL	NAKSHATRA	NANCY-MAY
NAIMUR	NAKUL	NANCY-RAE
NAINA	NALA	NANCY-ROSE
NAINIKA	NALA-MAE	NANDAN
NAINSI	NALA-ROSE	NANDANA
NAIOMI	NALAH	NANDI
NAIRA	NALAN	NANDIKA
NAIRAH	NALANI	NANDIN
NAISHA	NALEDI	NANDINI
NAISHE	NALI	NANDIPHA
NAITE	NALIN	NANDITA
NAITHAN	NALINI	NANDOR
NAITIK	NALISHA	NANETTE
NAIYA	NALY	NANKI
NAIYAH	NAM	NANNETTE
NAIYANA	NAMAAN	NANSI
NAJA	NAMAN	NANW
NAJAF	NAMEER	NAO
NAJAH	NAMEERA	NAOD
NAJAM	NAMIR	NAOISE
NAJAT	NAMIRA	NAOKI
NAJEEB	NAMIRAH	NAOME
NAJEEM	NAMISH	NAOMI
NAJI	NAMIT	NAOMI-ROSE
NAJIA	NAMITA	NAOMIE
NAJIAH	NAMO	NAPHTALI
NAJIB	NAMRA	NAQEEB
NAJIBA	NAMRAH	NAQIB
NAJIBAH	NAMRATA	NAQQASH
NAJIFA	NAMRITA	NAQUAN
NAJIIB	NAN	NARA
NAJIM	NANA	NARAIN
NAJIYAH	NANA-YAA	NARAYA
NAJLA	NANAK	NARAYAN
NAJMA	NANAKI	NARCIS
NAJMAH	NANAKO	NARCISA
NAJMIN	NANAMI	NARCISSE
NAJMO	NANCEE	NARDIA
NAJMUL	NANCEY	NARDOS
NAJWA	NANCI	NAREECE
NAKAI	NANCIE	NAREEN
NAKASH	NANCIE-MAI	NARELLE

NAREN	NASRI	NATASSIA
NARESH	NASRIN	NATASSJA
NARGAS	NASRIYA	NATASZA
NARGES	NASRUDIN	NATAYA
NARGIS	NASSAR	NATAYAH
NARIAH	NASSEM	NATE
NARIN	NASSER	NATEA
NARINDER	NASSIM	NATHALIA
NARISSA	NASSIR	NATHALIE
NARIYAH	NASSOR	NATHALY
NARJES	NASTAHO	NATHAN
NARJIS	NASTASSJA	NATHAN-JAMES
NARLA	NASTAZJA	NATHAN-LEE
NARMEEN	NASTEHA	NATHANAEL
NARMIN	NASTEHO	NATHANEAL
NARYAN	NASYA	NATHANEL
NASAR	NAT	NATHANIA
NASEEBA	NATACHA	NATHANIAL
NASEEHA	NATAHLIA	NATHANIEL
NASEEHAH	NATALEE	NATHANUAL
NASEEM	NATALI	NATHANUEL
NASEEMA	NATALIA	NATHASHA
NASEER	NATALIA-ROSE	NATHEN
NASEERAH	NATALIAH	NATHNAEL
NASER	NATALIE	NATHON
NASH	NATALIJA	NATISHA
NASHAD	NATALINA	NATNAEL
NASHARN	NATALIYA	NATSUKI
NASHAUN	NATALKA	NATSUMI
NASHAWN	NATALLIA	NAUFAL
NASHE	NATALLIE	NAUMAAN
NASHITA	NATALY	NAUMAN
NASHRA	NATALYA	NAUREEN
NASHWA	NATALYA-ROSE	NAURIS
NASHWAN	NATAN	NAUSHEEN
NASIA	NATANAEL	NAVA
NASIF	NATANEL	NAVAEH
NASIFAH	NATANIA	NAVARRO
NASIHA	NATANIEL	NAVAYA
NASIM	NATANYA	NAVAYAH
NASIMA	NATAS	NAVDEEP
NASIR	NATASA	NAVEAH
NASIRA	NATASCHA	NAVED
NASIRAH	NATASHA	NAVEED
NASMA	NATASHAH	NAVEEN
NASR	NATASHIA	NAVEENA
NASRA	NATASIA	NAVENA
NASREEN	NATASJA	NAVID

NAVIN	NAYLAA	NAZMIYE
NAVINA	NAYLAH	NAZMUL
NAVINDER	NAYLAN	NAZNEEN
NAVISHA	NAYLEN	NAZNIN
NAVJIT	NAYLOR	NAZREEN
NAVJOT	NAYM	NAZRIN
NAVKIRAT	NAYMA	NDEY
NAVLEEN	NAYNA	NDIDI
NAVNEET	NAYOMI	NE-YO
NAVPREET	NAYRA	NEA
NAVRAJ	NAYSA	NEAH
NAVREET	NAYSHA	NEAL
NAVROOP	NAYSHARN	NEALA
NAVTEJ	NAYTE	NEAMH
NAVY	NAYTHAN	NEAVE
NAVYA	NAYYAB	NEBI
NAWA	NAZ	NECATI
NAWAAL	NAZAHA	NECHAMA
NAWAB	NAZAM	NECO
NAWAF	NAZANEEN	NECTARIA
NAWAL	NAZANIN	NECTARIE
NAWAR	NAZAR	NED
NAWAZ	NAZARENE	NEDA
NAWEED	NAZARIY	NEDAL
NAWEL	NAZEEFA	NEDAS
NAWFAL	NAZEEFAH	NEDW
NAWID	NAZEEHA	NEEHA
NAYA	NAZEEM	NEEKA
NAYAAB	NAZEERA	NEEKO
NAYAB	NAZEERAH	NEEL
NAYAH	NAZIA	NEELA
NAYAN	NAZIAH	NEELAM
NAYANA	NAZIFA	NEELEY
NAYARA	NAZIFAH	NEELIMA
NAYEB	NAZIHA	NEELUM
NAYEEM	NAZIHAH	NEELY
NAYEEMA	NAZIM	NEEMA
NAYEEMUL	NAZIMA	NEEMAH
NAYEF	NAZIR	NEENA
NAYEL	NAZIRA	NEER
NAYELI	NAZIRAH	NEERAJ
NAYEM	NAZISH	NEERAV
NAYEMA	NAZLI	NEESA
NAYEN	NAZLICAN	NEESHA
NAYHA	NAZMA	NEESON
NAYIA	NAZMEEN	NEETI
NAYIM	NAZMIN	NEETU
NAYLA	NAZMINA	NEEV

NEEVA	NELLIE-MAY	NESRIN
NEEVAH	NELLIE-RAE	NESRINE
NEEVE	NELLIE-ROSE	NESSA
NEEYA	NELLY	NESTA
NEFELI	NELLY-RAE	NESTOR
NEFERTARI	NELLY-ROSE	NETANEL
NEFERTITI	NELSON	NETANYA
NEFES	NEMA	NETHAN
NEGAH	NEMANJA	NETHMI
NEGAN	NEMI	NETHRA
NEGAR	NEMO	NETRA
NEGIN	NEMUEL	NETTA
NEHA	NENA	NETTIE
NEHAAN	NENE	NEVA
NEHAL	NENEH	NEVAAN
NEHAN	NENYASHA	NEVADA
NEHARA	NEO	NEVAEH
NEHEMIAH	NEOLA	NEVAEH-FAITH
NEHIR	NEOMA	NEVAEH-GRACE
NEHMIA	NEOMI	NEVAEH-HOPE
NEIDAS	NEON	NEVAEH-LEIGH
NEIKO	NEONA	NEVAEH-LOUISE
NEIL	NEPHELE	NEVAEH-MAE
NEILA	NEPHELI	NEVAEH-MAI
NEILAN	NEPHTALIE	NEVAEH-MARIE
NEILAS	NERAYA	NEVAEH-MAY
NEILESH	NEREA	NEVAEH-RAE
NEILL	NERGIZ	NEVAEH-ROSE
NEIMA	NERI	NEVAEH-SKYE
NEIRIN	NERIA	NEVAEHA
NEISHA	NERIAH	NEVAN
NEITANAS	NERICE	NEVAYA
NEITAS	NERILE	NEVAYAH
NEITONAS	NERINE	NEVE
NEIVA	NERISSA	NEVEAH
NEIVE	NERISSE	NEVEN
NEKITA	NERIYA	NEVEYAH
NEKO	NERIYAH	NEVIAH
NEL	NERMIN	NEVIE
NELA	NERO	NEVILLE
NELI	NERYS	NEVIN
NELIA	NESE	NEVYN
NELL	NESHA	NEWTON
NELLA	NESIA	NEYA
NELLE	NESIAH	NEYAH
NELLI	NESLIHAN	NEYHA
NELLIE	NESMA	NEYLA
NELLIE-MAE	NESREEN	NEYLAN

NEYMAR
NEYO
NEYSA
NEZAR
NEZIAH
NGA
NGAIRE
NGOC
NGOZI
NGOZICHUKWU
NGOZICHUKWUKA
NGUYEN
NHI
NHYIRA
NIA
NIA-MAI
NIA-ROSE
NIAH
NIAL
NIALA
NIALAH
NIALL
NIALLE
NIAM
NIAMAH
NIAMBH
NIAMH
NIAMPH
NIAN
NIAOMI
NIARA
NIAV
NIAYA
NIAZ
NIBODH
NIBRAS
NICA
NICCI
NICCO
NICCOLO
NICHA
NICHELLE
NICHOL
NICHOLA
NICHOLAI
NICHOLAS
NICHOLE
NICHOLL

NICK
NICKEISHA
NICKI
NICKITA
NICKLAS
NICKO
NICKOLA
NICKOLAS
NICKOY
NICKSON
NICKY
NICLAS
NICO
NICODEM
NICODEMUS
NICOL
NICOLA
NICOLAAS
NICOLAE
NICOLAI
NICOLAS
NICOLE
NICOLE-LOUISE
NICOLETA
NICOLETTA
NICOLETTE
NICOLINA
NICOLL
NICOLLE
NICOLO
NICOS
NICOY
NIDA
NIDAA
NIDAH
NIDAL
NIDHA
NIDHI
NIEL
NIELS
NIEMA
NIENKE
NIESHA
NIEVE
NIFEMI
NIGEL
NIGELLA
NIHA

NIHAAL
NIHAD
NIHAL
NIHAN
NIHAR
NIHARIKA
NIHIRA
NII
NIK
NIKA
NIKAN
NIKAS
NIKASH
NIKAYA
NIKAYLA
NIKEISHA
NIKESH
NIKESHA
NIKET
NIKETA
NIKHIL
NIKHITA
NIKI
NIKIA
NIKIL
NIKINI
NIKISHA
NIKITA
NIKITAS
NIKITHA
NIKITTA
NIKIYA
NIKKALA
NIKKI
NIKKIA
NIKKITA
NIKKO
NIKLAS
NIKLAUS
NIKO
NIKODEM
NIKOL
NIKOLA
NIKOLAI
NIKOLAJ
NIKOLAOS
NIKOLAS
NIKOLASS

NIKOLAUS	NINO	NISHITA
NIKOLAY	NIOBE	NISHKA
NIKOLE	NIOMI	NISHMA
NIKOLETA	NIOMIE	NISHTA
NIKOLETT	NIR	NISHTHA
NIKOLETTA	NIRA	NISREEN
NIKOLIA	NIRAH	NISSA
NIKOLINA	NIRAJ	NISSI
NIKOLOZ	NIRAL	NITA
NIKOS	NIRALI	NITAI
NIKOU	NIRAN	NITARA
NIKS	NIRANJAN	NITASHA
NIKUL	NIRAV	NITESH
NIKUNJ	NIRBANI	NITHARSAN
NILA	NIRBHAY	NITHARSHAN
NILAH	NIREL	NITHILA
NILAN	NIRMA	NITHIN
NILANI	NIRMAL	NITHISH
NILAY	NIRMIT	NITHUSH
NILE	NIROSHAN	NITHUSHA
NILEEMA	NIRUJA	NITHUSHAN
NILES	NIRUJAN	NITHYA
NILESH	NIRUSHAN	NITI
NILIMA	NIRVAAN	NITIKA
NILOFAR	NIRVAIR	NITIN
NILOOFAR	NIRVAN	NITYA
NILS	NIRVANA	NIUSHA
NILSU	NIRVI	NIV
NILUFAR	NISA	NIVA
NILUFER	NISANUR	NIVAAN
NIMA	NISAR	NIVAN
NIMAH	NISARG	NIVEA
NIMAO	NISBA	NIVEDHA
NIMAT	NISBAH	NIVEN
NIMCO	NISCHAL	NIVETHA
NIMESH	NISHA	NIVETHAN
NIMISHA	NISHAAN	NIVIN
NIMO	NISHAAT	NIVISHA
NIMRA	NISHAD	NIXIE
NIMRAH	NISHAL	NIXON
NIMRAT	NISHAN	NIYA
NIMRATA	NISHANT	NIYAH
NIMRIT	NISHAT	NIYAM
NIMRITA	NISHATH	NIYAN
NIMROD	NISHCHAL	NIYANA
NIMUE	NISHI	NIYAT
NINA	NISHIKA	NIYATI
NINIOLA	NISHIL	NIYAZ

NIYEMA
NIYLA
NIYLAH
NIZAM
NIZAMUDDIN
NIZAMUL
NIZAR
NJ
NJERI
NKECHI
NKEMDILIM
NKOSI
NMA
NNAEMEKA
NNAMDI
NNANNA
NNEKA
NNENNA
NNEOMA
NOA
NOAH
NOAH-GEORGE
NOAH-JACK
NOAH-JAMES
NOAH-JAY
NOAH-JOHN
NOAH-LEE
NOAM
NOAMAN
NOAMI
NOAN
NOAR
NOBEL
NOBLE
NOE
NOEL
NOELA
NOELANI
NOELIA
NOELLA
NOELLE
NOEMI
NOEMIE
NOH
NOHA
NOJUS
NOKUTENDA
NOL

NOLA
NOLAH
NOLAN
NOLAWI
NOLEN
NOLWENN
NOMAAN
NOMAN
NOMI
NOMIN
NOMSA
NON
NONA
NOOH
NOOMI
NOON
NOOR
NOOR-AL-AIN
NOOR-FATIMA
NOOR-UL-AIN
NOOR-UL-HUDA
NOORA
NOORAH
NOORAIN
NOORAN
NOORDIN
NOORI
NOORIA
NOORIYA
NOORIYAH
NOORJAHAN
NOORUL
NOORULAIN
NOR
NORA
NORAH
NORAIZ
NORBERT
NOREEN
NORI
NORIK
NORINA
NORMA
NORMAN
NORRIS
NORSEEN
NORTH
NORTON

NOSAKHARE
NOSHABA
NOSHEEN
NOSHIN
NOSSON
NOTHANDO
NOUF
NOUH
NOUMAAN
NOUMAN
NOUR
NOURA
NOURAH
NOURAN
NOUREDDINE
NOUREEN
NOURHAN
NOURIA
NOURIN
NOUSHIN
NOVA
NOVA-LEE
NOVAH
NOVAK
NOVALEE
NOVELLA
NOWSHIN
NOYA
NOYAN
NOZOMI
NTANDOYENKOSI
NUALA
NUAYM
NUAYMAH
NUBAID
NUBIA
NUH
NUHA
NUHAA
NUJHAT
NULA
NUMA
NUMAAN
NUMAIR
NUMAN
NUMAYR
NUMRA
NUNO

NUO	NYELA
NUR	NYELLA
NURA	NYEMA
NURADIN	NYESHA
NURAH	NYIAH
NURAIZ	NYIEMA
NURALAIN	NYIMA
NURAN	NYIMAH
NURAT	NYLA
NURAY	NYLA-RAE
NURAZ	NYLA-ROSE
NURDIN	NYLAH
NUREEN	NYLAH-RAE
NUREIN	NYLAH-ROSE
NURETTIN	NYLE
NURI	NYLES
NURIA	NYNKE
NURIN	NYOMI
NURIYA	NYRA
NURIYAH	NYRAH
NURUDDIN	NYREE
NURUL	NYRON
NUSAIBA	NYSA
NUSAIBAH	NYSHA
NUSAIYBAH	NYSSA
NUSAYBA	NYX
NUSAYBAH	NZA
NUSEYBA	
NUSHRAT	
NUSRAT	
NUSRATH	
NUUH	
NUVEE	
NUWAIR	
NUWAIRA	
NUZHA	
NUZHAT	
NYA	
NYAH	
NYAL	
NYALL	
NYAN	
NYARA	
NYARAI	
NYASHA	
NYASIA	
NYE	
NYEESHA	

O

O'NEIL
O'NEILL
O'SHAE
O'SHAI
O'SHANE
O'SHAY
O'SHEA
OAK
OAKLAN
OAKLEA
OAKLEE
OAKLEIGH
OAKLEN
OAKLEY
OAKLEY-BLUE
OAKLEY-JAMES
OAKLEY-JAY
OAKLIE
OAKLY
OAKLYN
OANA
OASIS
OBADIAH
OBAFEMI
OBAID
OBAIDULLAH
OBALOLUWA
OBAN
OBED
OBEHI
OBERON
OBI
OBIAJULU
OBIANUJU
OBIE
OBINNA
OBIORA
OBY
OCEA
OCEAN
OCEAN-BLU
OCEAN-ROSE
OCEANA
OCEANE
OCEANIA
OCEANNA
OCEANNE
OCTAVE
OCTAVIA
OCTAVIAN
OCTAVIO
OCTAVIUS
ODAFE
ODELIA
ODELYA
ODEN
ODERA
ODESSA
ODETTA
ODETTE
ODHRAN
ODILE
ODILIA
ODIN
ODINAKACHUKWU
ODRIJA
ODUNAYO
ODYSSEAS
ODYSSEUS
OENONE
OFELIA
OFURE
OGECHI
OGECHUKWU
OGHENEBRUME
OGHENEFEGA
OGHENEFEJIRO
OGHENEMARO
OGHENEMINE
OGHENERUKEVWE
OGHENERUNO
OGHENETEGA
OGHENETEJIRI
OGHOSA
OGOCHUKWU
OGULCAN
OGUZ
OGUZHAN
OHANA
OHEMAA
OHENE
OHENEBA
OISIN
OJAS
OJASVI
OJAY
OKAN
OKECHUKWU
OKIKIOLA
OKKES
OKSANA
OKTAWIA
OKTAWIAN
OKTAY
OLA
OLABISI
OLABODE
OLACHI
OLADAPO
OLADAYO
OLADELE
OLADIMEJI
OLADIPO
OLADIPUPO
OLAEDO
OLAF
OLAITAN
OLAJIDE
OLAJUMOKE
OLAJUWON
OLAKUNLE
OLALEKAN
OLAMIDE
OLAMILEKAN
OLAMIPOSI
OLAN
OLANNA
OLANREWAJU
OLAOLUWA
OLAOLUWAKITAN
OLAREWAJU
OLASENI
OLASUBOMI
OLATAYO
OLATOKUNBO
OLATOMIWA
OLATUNBOSUN
OLATUNDE
OLATUNJI
OLAWALE

OLAYEMI
OLAYINKA
OLE
OLEG
OLEK
OLENA
OLENKA
OLESIA
OLESYA
OLGA
OLGIERD
OLI
OLIE
OLIMPIA
OLIN
OLINA
OLISAEMEKA
OLIUR
OLIVA
OLIVE
OLIVE-ROSE
OLIVEA
OLIVER
OLIVER-DANIEL
OLIVER-GEORGE
OLIVER-JACK
OLIVER-JAMES
OLIVER-JAY
OLIVER-JOHN
OLIVER-LEE
OLIVERIS
OLIVERS
OLIVIA
OLIVIA-
OLIVIA-ANN
OLIVIA-FAITH
OLIVIA-GRACE
OLIVIA-HOPE
OLIVIA-JADE
OLIVIA-JANE
OLIVIA-JAYNE
OLIVIA-JEAN
OLIVIA-JO
OLIVIA-LEA
OLIVIA-LEE
OLIVIA-LEIGH
OLIVIA-LILLY
OLIVIA-LILY

OLIVIA-LOUISE
OLIVIA-MAE
OLIVIA-MAI
OLIVIA-MARIE
OLIVIA-MAY
OLIVIA-PAIGE
OLIVIA-RAE
OLIVIA-ROSE
OLIVIAH
OLIVIER
OLIVIJA
OLIVYA
OLIWER
OLIWIA
OLIWIER
OLLE
OLLEY
OLLI
OLLIE
OLLIE-JAI
OLLIE-JAMES
OLLIE-JAY
OLLIE-JOE
OLLIE-RAY
OLLIVER
OLLY
OLLY-JAMES
OLLY-JAY
OLLY-RAY
OLOLADE
OLORUNTOBA
OLSA
OLSEN
OLSI
OLT
OLTA
OLTI
OLTION
OLUBUKOLA
OLUBUNMI
OLUCHI
OLUFEMI
OLUFUNKE
OLUFUNMILAYO
OLUFUNMILOLA
OLUGBENGA
OLUJIMI
OLUKAYODE

OLUKEMI
OLUMAYOWA
OLUMIDE
OLUMUYIWA
OLUROTIMI
OLUSEGUN
OLUSEUN
OLUSEYI
OLUSOLA
OLUTOBI
OLUTOMI
OLUTOMILOLA
OLUTOYIN
OLUWABUKOLA
OLUWABUKUNMI
OLUWABUSAYOMI
OLUWADABIRA
OLUWADAMILARE
OLUWADAMILOJU
OLUWADAMILOLA
OLUWADAMISI
OLUWADARA
OLUWADARASIMI
OLUWADARE
OLUWADEMILADE
OLUWADOLAPO
OLUWADUNMININU
OLUWADUROTIMI
OLUWAFEMI
OLUWAFERANMI
OLUWAFEYIKEMI
OLUWAFIFEHANMI
OLUWAFIKAYO
OLUWAFIKAYOMI
OLUWAFIKUNAYOMI
OLUWAFIKUNMI
OLUWAFISAYO
OLUWAFISAYOMI
OLUWAFOLABOMI
OLUWAFOLAJIMI
OLUWAFOLAKEMI
OLUWAFUNMILAYO
OLUWAFUNMILOLA
OLUWAFUNTAN
OLUWAGBEMIGA
OLUWAGBEMISOLA
OLUWAGBENGA
OLUWAJOBA

OLUWAJOMILOJU
OLUWAJUWON
OLUWAJUWONLO
OLUWAKANYINSOLA
OLUWAKAYODE
OLUWAKEMI
OLUWAKOREDE
OLUWALAYOMI
OLUWALONIMI
OLUWAMAYOMIKUN
OLUWAMAYOWA
OLUWAMUYIWA
OLUWANIFEMI
OLUWAPELUMI
OLUWAREMILEKUN
OLUWAROTIMI
OLUWASEGUN
OLUWASEMILORE
OLUWASEUN
OLUWASEYI
OLUWASEYIFUNMI
OLUWASEYITAN
OLUWASHINAYOMI
OLUWASHINDARA
OLUWASHOLA
OLUWASIJIBOMI
OLUWASOLA
OLUWATAMILORE
OLUWATARAMISORE
OLUWATENIAYO
OLUWATENIOLA
OLUWATIMILEHIN
OLUWATIMILEYIN
OLUWATISE
OLUWATISHE
OLUWATOBA
OLUWATOBI
OLUWATOBILOBA
OLUWATOFUNMI
OLUWATOMI
OLUWATOMILOLA
OLUWATOMISIN
OLUWATOMIWA
OLUWATONI
OLUWATONILOBA
OLUWATOSIN
OLUWATOYIN
OLUWATOYOSI

OLUWATUMININU
OLUWATUNMISE
OLUWAYEMISI
OLUWOLE
OLUYEMI
OLWEN
OLWETHU
OLWYN
OLY
OLYMPIA
OLYVIA
OM
OMAAN
OMAID
OMAIMA
OMAIR
OMAIRA
OMAMA
OMAN
OMAR
OMARA
OMARI
OMARIAN
OMARIE
OMARIO
OMARION
OMAYA
OMAYMA
OMAYR
OMED
OMEGA
OMER
OMERA
OMI
OMID
OMISHA
OMKAR
OMNIA
OMOBOLAJI
OMOBOLANLE
OMOLABAKE
OMOLADE
OMOLARA
OMOLAYO
OMOLOLA
OMORINSOLA
OMOSEDE
OMOTARA

OMOTAYO
OMOTOLA
OMOTOLANI
OMOTOYOSI
OMOWONUOLA
OMOWUNMI
OMRAN
OMRI
ONA
ONAJITE
ONAYA
ONDER
ONDREJ
ONEIL
ONELI
ONI
ONIAS
ONIKA
ONKAR
ONNI
ONOME
ONORA
ONOSETALE
ONUR
ONYEBUCHI
ONYEDIKACHI
ONYEKACHI
ONYEKACHUKWU
ONYINYE
ONYINYECHI
ONYINYECHUKWU
ONYX
OONA
OONAGH
OPAL
OPEMIPO
OPEOLUWA
OPEYEMI
OPHELIA
OPHELIA-ROSE
OPHELIE
OPIE
OPRAH
OR
ORA
ORACLE
ORAN
ORCHID

ORELIA	ORNELA	OSHEA
OREN	ORNELLA	OSHER
OREOFEOLUWA	OROBOSA	OSHI
OREOLUWA	ORPHEUS	OSHIAN
OREST	ORRAN	OSHUN
ORESTAS	ORREN	OSIAN
ORESTIS	ORRIE	OSIAN-LEE
ORFEAS	ORRIN	OSIAS
ORGES	ORRY	OSINACHI
ORGESA	ORRYN	OSIRIS
ORGITO	ORSEN	OSKA
ORHAN	ORSON	OSKAR
ORI	ORVILLE	OSKARAS
ORIAH	OSAAMA	OSKARS
ORIAN	OSAGIE	OSKER
ORIANA	OSAHENRUMWEN	OSLO
ORIANE	OSAHON	OSMAN
ORIANNA	OSAMA	OSOB
ORIANNE	OSAMAH	OSSAMA
ORIANTHI	OSAMUDIAMEN	OSSIAN
ORIEL	OSARETIN	OSSIE
ORIELLA	OSARIEMEN	OSTARA
ORIELLE	OSARO	OSTEN
ORIN	OSARUGUE	OSTIN
ORINTA	OSASERE	OSTYN
ORION	OSAYANDE	OSWALD
ORISSA	OSAYUWAMEN	OSWIN
ORITSE	OSAZE	OSZKAR
ORLA	OSAZEE	OTAVIO
ORLA-FAITH	OSAZUWA	OTHMAN
ORLA-GRACE	OSBERT	OTHNIEL
ORLA-MAE	OSBORN	OTILIA
ORLA-RAE	OSBORNE	OTIS
ORLA-ROSE	OSBOURNE	OTNIEL
ORLAGH	OSCA	OTO
ORLAH	OSCAR	OTSO
ORLAIGH	OSCAR-GEORGE	OTTALIE
ORLAITH	OSCAR-JACK	OTTAVIO
ORLAN	OSCAR-JAI	OTTER
ORLANA	OSCAR-JAMES	OTTILIA
ORLAND	OSCAR-JAY	OTTILIE
ORLANDA	OSCAR-LEE	OTTIS
ORLANDO	OSCAR-THOMAS	OTTO
ORLEY	OSEI	OTTOLINE
ORLI	OSGAR	OTYLIA
ORLIN	OSHAE	OUMAR
ORLY	OSHAN	OUMIE
ORNA	OSHANE	OUMOU

OUSAINOU
OUSAMA
OUSMAN
OUSMANE
OUSSAMA
OVI
OVIE
OVIYA
OVIYAN
OWAIN
OWAIS
OWAN
OWEN
OWEN-JAMES
OWENA
OWI
OWIN
OWURA
OWYN
OWYNN
OYINADE
OYINDAMOLA
OYINKANSOLA
OYINLOLA
OYKU
OZ
OZAIR
OZAN
OZCAN
OZGE
OZGUR
OZIAS
OZIL
OZIOMA
OZKAN
OZLEM
OZWALD
OZZI
OZZIE
OZZY

P

PA
PAA
PAAPA
PAARTH
PAAVAN
PAAVANA
PAAYAL
PABLO
PACEY
PACHA
PADDY
PADME
PADRAIC
PADRAIG
PAGAN
PAGE
PAGEN
PAHAL
PAIGAN
PAIGE
PAIGE-LEIGH
PAIGE-LOUISE
PAIGE-MARIE
PAIGE-ROSE
PAIGEN
PAIGHTON
PAIGNTON
PAIGTON
PAIJE
PAISLEA
PAISLEE
PAISLEIGH
PAISLEY
PAISLEY-GRACE
PAISLEY-MAE
PAISLEY-MAI
PAISLEY-MAY
PAISLEY-RAE
PAISLEY-ROSE
PAITON
PAITYN
PAK
PAKEEZA
PAKEEZAH

PAL
PALAK
PALESA
PALLAVI
PALMER
PALOMA
PALVI
PALVINDER
PALWASHA
PAMELA
PAMELLA
PANA
PANAGIOTIS
PANASHE
PANAV
PANAYIOTA
PANAYIOTIS
PANAYOTIS
PANDORA
PANIZ
PANKA
PANNA
PANSY
PANTH
PAOLA
PAOLO
PAPA
PAPE
PARADISE
PARAM
PARAMVEER
PARAMVIR
PARAN
PARAS
PARASKEVI
PARDEEP
PAREESA
PARHAM
PARI
PARIA
PARICE
PARIDHI
PARIN
PARINA
PARINAZ
PARINEET
PARINITA
PARIS

PARIS-LEIGH
PARISA
PARISE
PARISH
PARISHA
PARISHAY
PARISHI
PARISS
PARISSA
PARISSE
PARIZA
PARKER
PARKER-JAMES
PARKER-ROSE
PARLEEN
PARMEET
PARMIDA
PARMINDER
PARMIS
PARMVEER
PARMVIR
PARNEET
PARNIKA
PARRIS
PARSA
PARTH
PARTHA
PARTHIV
PARUL
PARVATHI
PARVATI
PARVEEN
PARVESH
PARVEZ
PARVIN
PARVINA
PARVINDER
PARYA
PARYS
PASCAL
PASCALE
PASCHA
PASHA
PASQUALE
PASSION
PATIENCE
PATRIC
PATRICE

PATRICIA	PAWAN	PENG
PATRICIJA	PAWANDEEP	PENIEL
PATRICIO	PAWEL	PENINA
PATRICK	PAX	PENN
PATRIK	PAXTON	PENNIE
PATRIKAS	PAYAL	PENNY
PATRIKS	PAYAM	PENNY-MAE
PATRISIA	PAYGE	PENNY-MAY
PATRYCJA	PAYNTON	PENNY-ROSE
PATRYK	PAYSON	PENUEL
PATSIE	PAYTEN	PEONY
PATSY	PAYTON	PEPE
PATTI	PAYTON-GRACE	PEPPER
PAU	PAYTON-LEIGH	PERAN
PAUL	PAYVIN	PERCIVAL
PAUL-JUNIOR	PAYWAND	PERCY
PAULA	PAZ	PERDITA
PAULETTE	PEACE	PERDY
PAULIE	PEACH	PEREGRIN
PAULINA	PEACHES	PEREGRINE
PAULINE	PEARCE	PEREL
PAULIUS	PEARL	PEREZ
PAULO	PEARL-ROSE	PERI
PAULS	PEARLA	PERIHAN
PAVAN	PEARLE	PERL
PAVANDEEP	PEARSE	PERLA
PAVANI	PEARSON	PERLE
PAVANJIT	PEBBLES	PERNELL
PAVANVEER	PEDRAM	PEROLA
PAVANVIR	PEDRO	PERPETUA
PAVEL	PEER	PERRAN
PAVENDEEP	PEGGIE	PERRI
PAVIN	PEGGY	PERRIE
PAVINDER	PEGGY-MAE	PERRIE-ROSE
PAVISH	PEI	PERRIN
PAVISHAN	PEIGHTON	PERRY
PAVIT	PEIQI	PERSEPHONE
PAVITAR	PELAGIA	PERSEPHONIE
PAVITH	PELAYO	PERSEUS
PAVITHRA	PELE	PERSIA
PAVLE	PELHAM	PERSIS
PAVLEEN	PELIN	PESSY
PAVLINA	PELLE	PETA
PAVLO	PEMA	PETAL
PAVLOS	PEMBE	PETAR
PAVNEET	PENDA	PETE
PAVNI	PENELOPE	PETEK
PAVOL	PENELOPE-ROSE	PETER

PETER-JAMES	PHILLIPPA	PINCHOS
PETER-JUNIOR	PHILOMENA	PIO
PETR	PHINEAS	PIOTR
PETRA	PHINEHAS	PIOUS
PETRAS	PHINN	PIP
PETRINA	PHINNAEUS	PIPER
PETROS	PHOEBE	PIPER-MARIE
PETRU	PHOEBE-	PIPER-RAE
PETRUS	PHOEBE-ANN	PIPER-ROSE
PETRUTA	PHOEBE-GRACE	PIPPA
PEYTON	PHOEBE-JANE	PIPPA-LEIGH
PEYTON-LEIGH	PHOEBE-JAYNE	PIPPA-LOUISE
PEYTON-LOUISE	PHOEBE-JO	PIPPA-MAE
PEYTON-ROSE	PHOEBE-LEE	PIPPA-ROSE
PHAEDRA	PHOEBE-LEIGH	PIPPI
PHANUEL	PHOEBE-LOU	PIPPIN
PHARAOH	PHOEBE-LOUISE	PIR
PHARELL	PHOEBE-MAE	PIRAN
PHARELLE	PHOEBE-MAI	PIRANAVAN
PHAREZ	PHOEBE-MARIE	PIRAVEEN
PHARIS	PHOEBE-MAY	PIRAVEENA
PHARREL	PHOEBE-RAE	PIRRAN
PHARRELL	PHOEBE-ROSE	PIUS
PHARREN	PHOEBIE	PIXI
PHAT	PHOENIX	PIXIE
PHEBE	PHOENIX-ROSE	PIXIE-BEAU
PHEBEE	PHOENYX	PIXIE-BELLE
PHELAN	PHOIBE	PIXIE-LEIGH
PHELIM	PHONG	PIXIE-LOU
PHELIX	PHUONG	PIXIE-MAE
PHENIX	PHYLLIDA	PIXIE-RAE
PHEOBE	PHYLLIS	PIXIE-ROSE
PHEOBE-ANN	PIA	PIYA
PHEOBIE	PIERCE	PIYUSH
PHEONIX	PIERLUIGI	PJ
PHI	PIERO	PLAMEDI
PHIA	PIERRE	PLAMEN
PHIL	PIERS	PLAMENA
PHILBERT	PIERSE	PLATON
PHILEMON	PIERSON	PLUM
PHILIP	PIETER	POLA
PHILIPA	PIETRA	POLAT
PHILIPP	PIETRO	POLINA
PHILIPPA	PIHU	POLLIE
PHILIPPE	PIJUS	POLLY
PHILIPPOS	PILAR	POLLY-ANNA
PHILLIP	PINAR	POLLY-MAE
PHILLIPA	PINCHAS	POLLY-ROSE

POLLYANNA	PORSHIA	PRANIT
POOJA	PORTER	PRANITA
POONAM	PORTIA	PRANITH
POPI	POSEY	PRANITHA
POPPI	POSIE	PRANJAL
POPPIE	POSY	PRANSHI
POPPIE-ANN	POYRAZ	PRANSHU
POPPIE-LEIGH	PRABAL	PRANSI
POPPIE-MAE	PRABDEEP	PRAPTI
POPPIE-MAI	PRABH	PRARTHANA
POPPIE-RAE	PRABHDEEP	PRASANNA
POPPIE-ROSE	PRABHGUN	PRASHANT
POPPY	PRABHJEET	PRATEEK
POPPY-ANN	PRABHJOT	PRATHAM
POPPY-ANNE	PRABHKIRAT	PRATHANA
POPPY-BELLE	PRABHLEEN	PRATIK
POPPY-ELIZABETH	PRABHNOOR	PRATYUSH
POPPY-ELLA	PRABHREET	PRAVAN
POPPY-GRACE	PRABHROOP	PRAVEEN
POPPY-ISABELLA	PRABHVEER	PRAVEENA
POPPY-JANE	PRABHVIR	PRAVEER
POPPY-JAY	PRABJOT	PRAVIN
POPPY-JAYNE	PRABLEEN	PRAVINA
POPPY-JEAN	PRABVEER	PRAVLEEN
POPPY-JO	PRACHI	PRAYAAG
POPPY-LEA	PRADEEP	PRAYAG
POPPY-LEE	PRADYUN	PRAYAN
POPPY-LEIGH	PRAGATI	PRECILIA
POPPY-LOU	PRAISE	PRECIOUS
POPPY-LOUISE	PRAJIN	PREENA
POPPY-MAE	PRAJIT	PREESHA
POPPY-MAI	PRAJNA	PREET
POPPY-MARIE	PRAJWAL	PREETHIKA
POPPY-MAY	PRAKASH	PREETHY
POPPY-RAE	PRAKRITI	PREETI
POPPY-ROSE	PRANALI	PREEYA
POPPY-SUE	PRANATI	PREHAAN
POPPY-WILLOW	PRANAV	PREKSHA
POPPYROSE	PRANAVAN	PREM
PORCHA	PRANAVI	PREMAL
PORCHIA	PRANAY	PRENTICE
PORCIA	PRANAYA	PRERANA
PORSCHA	PRANEEL	PRERNA
PORSCHE	PRANEET	PRESHA
PORSCHE-LEIGH	PRANEIL	PRESLAV
PORSHA	PRANESH	PRESLAVA
PORSHA-LEIGH	PRANIKA	PRESLEY
PORSHA-MARIE	PRANISH	PRESTEN

PRESTON
PRESTON-JAMES
PRESTON-LEE
PRESTYN
PRETTY
PREYA
PREZLEY
PRIA
PRIAM
PRIANKA
PRICILLA
PRIMROSE
PRINA
PRINCE
PRINCESS
PRINCETON
PRINCEWILL
PRINCY
PRISCA
PRISCILA
PRISCILLA
PRISCILLA-ROSE
PRISEIS
PRISH
PRISHA
PRITAM
PRITESH
PRITHA
PRITHIKA
PRITHVI
PRITHVIRAJ
PRITI
PRITIKA
PRITPAL
PRIYA
PRIYA-ROSE
PRIYAA
PRIYAH
PRIYAL
PRIYAM
PRIYAN
PRIYANA
PRIYANK
PRIYANKA
PRIYANSH
PRIYANSHI
PRIYANSHU
PRIYASHA

PRIYEN
PRIYESH
PROMISE
PROSPER
PRUDENCE
PRUE
PRUSHA
PRYCE
PRYS
PRZEMYSLAW
PSALM
PTOLEMY
PUI
PUJA
PUJAN
PUNEET
PUNIT
PURAN
PURAV
PURDEY
PURDY
PURITY
PURVA
PURVI
PUTERI
PYPER

Q

QAASIM
QADAR
QADEER
QADIR
QAILAH
QAIM
QAIS
QAISER
QAMAR
QASAM
QASID
QASIM
QASSIM
QASWA
QAYLAH
QAYS
QAYYIM
QAZI
QENDRESA
QENDRIM
QI
QIAN
QIAO
QIN
QING
QIRAAT
QIRAT
QUADE
QUAID
QUAN
QUANG
QUASIM
QUAZI
QUDSIA
QUDSIYAH
QUDUS
QUEEN
QUEENIE
QUENTIN
QUERIDA
QUIANA
QUIANNA
QUILLAN
QUIN
QUINCEY
QUINCY
QUINLAN
QUINLEY
QUINN
QUINNE
QUINTEN
QUINTIN
QUINTON
QUINTUS
QUOC
QUORRA
QURATULAIN
QURRATUL
QUSAI
QUSAY
QUYNH

R

RA'EES
RA'EESAH
RA'ID
RA'NELL
RAABIA
RAABIAH
RAABIYA
RAADHIYA
RAADHIYAH
RAADIYA
RAADIYAH
RAAFAY
RAAFE
RAAFI
RAAGA
RAAHI
RAAHIL
RAAHIM
RAAHIMA
RAAHUL
RAAID
RAAINA
RAAJ
RAAJAN
RAAJVEER
RAAKHI
RAAM
RAAMEEN
RAANIA
RAANIYA
RAAVI
RAAYA
RAAYAN
RAAZIA
RAB
RABAB
RABAH
RABAIL
RABBI
RABBIA
RABEEA
RABEEAH
RABEYA
RABI

RABIA
RABIAH
RABIATOU
RABIHA
RABINA
RABIYA
RABIYAH
RABYA
RACHAEL
RACHAL
RACHANA
RACHEAL
RACHEL
RACHEL-LOUISE
RACHELE
RACHELL
RACHELLE
RACHID
RACHIT
RACHNA
RACIM
RACINE
RACQUEL
RADA
RADEK
RADEYAH
RADHA
RADHIA
RADHIKA
RADHIYA
RADI
RADIA
RADIKA
RADIN
RADIYA
RADIYAH
RADLEY
RADMAN
RADOMIR
RADOSLAV
RADOSLAVA
RADOSLAW
RADOST
RADU
RADVIN
RADWA
RADWAN
RADYAH

RAE
RAE-ANN
RAE-ANNE
RAEA
RAEANNA
RAEANNE
RAED
RAEED
RAEEF
RAEES
RAEESA
RAEESAH
RAEESE
RAEF
RAEFE
RAEGAN
RAEIS
RAEKWON
RAEL
RAELLE
RAEM
RAENA
RAENE
RAEON
RAEPH
RAEVEN
RAEWYN
RAEYA
RAF
RAFA
RAFAAN
RAFAEL
RAFAELA
RAFAELE
RAFAELLA
RAFAELS
RAFAL
RAFAN
RAFAT
RAFAY
RAFE
RAFEE
RAFEEF
RAFEH
RAFEL
RAFF
RAFFAEL
RAFFAELA

RAFFAELE
RAFFAELLA
RAFFAELLO
RAFFE
RAFFERTY
RAFFEY
RAFFI
RAFFY
RAFI
RAFIA
RAFIAH
RAFIAT
RAFID
RAFIDA
RAFIF
RAFIK
RAFIQ
RAFIUL
RAFSAN
RAGAD
RAGAN
RAGAVI
RAGEN
RAGHAD
RAGHAV
RAGHIB
RAGNAR
RAGUL
RAHA
RAHAAN
RAHAF
RAHAIL
RAHAN
RAHANA
RAHAND
RAHAT
RAHATH
RAHBIA
RAHEEB
RAHEEL
RAHEELA
RAHEEM
RAHEEMA
RAHEEMAH
RAHEEN
RAHEES
RAHEESA
RAHEIM

RAHEL
RAHELA
RAHEMA
RAHENA
RAHI
RAHIB
RAHID
RAHIEM
RAHIIMA
RAHIL
RAHILA
RAHIM
RAHIMA
RAHIMAH
RAHIN
RAHINA
RAHMA
RAHMAAN
RAHMAH
RAHMAN
RAHMAT
RAHMEEN
RAHMEL
RAHMO
RAHMONE
RAHOUL
RAHSAAN
RAHUL
RAHWA
RAI
RAIA
RAIAH
RAIAN
RAID
RAIDA
RAIDAH
RAIDEN
RAIENS
RAIF
RAIFAH
RAIFE
RAIGAN
RAIHA
RAIHAAN
RAIHAANAH
RAIHAN
RAIHANA
RAIMA

RAIMAH
RAIMONDS
RAIN
RAINA
RAINBOW
RAINE
RAINER
RAINEY
RAINIE
RAIS
RAISA
RAISAH
RAISHA
RAISSA
RAISY
RAITH
RAIVEER
RAIVO
RAIYA
RAIYAAN
RAIYAH
RAIYAN
RAIZEL
RAIZY
RAJ
RAJA
RAJAB
RAJAH
RAJAN
RAJANA
RAJANDEEP
RAJAT
RAJBIR
RAJDEEP
RAJEEV
RAJEN
RAJESH
RAJI
RAJIB
RAJINA
RAJINDER
RAJIV
RAJKUMAR
RAJMINA
RAJNA
RAJNEET
RAJNI
RAJPAL

RAJPREET
RAJU
RAJUN
RAJVEER
RAJVI
RAJVINDER
RAJVIR
RAJWINDER
RAKAI
RAKAN
RAKAYA
RAKEB
RAKEEB
RAKEEM
RAKESH
RAKHEE
RAKHI
RAKIB
RAKIBUR
RAKIM
RAKIN
RAKIYA
RAKIYAH
RAKSHA
RAKSHAN
RAKSHANA
RAKULAN
RALEIGH
RALF
RALFIE
RALFS
RALIAT
RALITSA
RALPH
RALPHI
RALPHIE
RALPHY
RALPHY-LEE
RALUCA
RAM
RAMA
RAMADAN
RAMAE
RAMAH
RAMAL
RAMAN
RAMANA
RAMANDEEP
RAMANI
RAMANPREET
RAMARI
RAMARIO
RAMARNI
RAMATOULIE
RAMATU
RAMATULAI
RAMAYA
RAMAZAN
RAMEEN
RAMEESA
RAMEESAH
RAMEESHA
RAMEEZ
RAMEEZA
RAMEL
RAMELL
RAMELLE
RAMESH
RAMESHA
RAMEY
RAMEZ
RAMI
RAMIA
RAMIAH
RAMILA
RAMIN
RAMINA
RAMINTA
RAMIR
RAMIREZ
RAMIRO
RAMIS
RAMISA
RAMISHA
RAMIYAH
RAMIZ
RAMLA
RAMLAH
RAMNEEK
RAMNEET
RAMNIK
RAMON
RAMONA
RAMONE
RAMSAY
RAMSEY
RAMSHA
RAMSHAH
RAMTIN
RAMY
RAMYA
RAMYAR
RAMZAN
RAMZI
RAMZY
RANA
RANAE
RANBIR
RAND
RANDA
RANDAL
RANDALL
RANDEEP
RANDELL
RANDOLPH
RANDY
RANEE
RANEEM
RANEL
RANELL
RANI
RANIA
RANIYA
RANIYAH
RANJEET
RANJIT
RANJODH
RANJOT
RANNA
RANULF
RANULPH
RANVEER
RANVIR
RANYA
RANYAH
RAO
RAOUF
RAOUL
RAPHA
RAPHAEL
RAPHAELA
RAPHAELLA
RAPHAELLE
RAPHEAL

RAPHEL	RAUNAK	RAYEES
RAQEEB	RAURI	RAYEN
RAQIB	RAUSHAN	RAYGAN
RAQIYA	RAVDEEP	RAYHA
RAQUEL	RAVEEN	RAYHAAN
RARES	RAVEENA	RAYHAN
RARESH	RAVEL	RAYHANA
RAS	RAVEN	RAYHANAH
RASA	RAVENNA	RAYIRTH
RASAN	RAVI	RAYLAN
RASEEL	RAVIN	RAYLEIGH
RASHA	RAVINA	RAYMON
RASHAAD	RAVINDER	RAYMOND
RASHAAN	RAVJOT	RAYMUND
RASHAD	RAVLEEN	RAYN
RASHAN	RAVNEET	RAYNA
RASHANA	RAVREET	RAYNARD
RASHANE	RAVZA	RAYNE
RASHARD	RAWA	RAYNIE
RASHARN	RAWAAN	RAYNOR
RASHAUN	RAWAD	RAYON
RASHAWN	RAWAN	RAYSA
RASHED	RAWAND	RAYSHAWN
RASHEDA	RAWAZ	RAYSSA
RASHEED	RAWDA	RAYVEN
RASHEEDA	RAWDAH	RAYVON
RASHEEDAT	RAWDHA	RAYYA
RASHEL	RAWDON	RAYYAAN
RASHI	RAWEN	RAYYAH
RASHID	RAWIA	RAYYAN
RASHIDA	RAY	RAYYANA
RASHIDAT	RAYA	RAZ
RASHIKA	RAYA-MAE	RAZA
RASHMA	RAYAAN	RAZAAN
RASHMI	RAYAH	RAZAN
RASHMIKA	RAYAN	RAZANE
RASIKA	RAYANA	RAZANNE
RASIM	RAYANE	RAZEEN
RASMUS	RAYANN	RAZEENA
RASNA	RAYANNA	RAZEENAH
RASTISLAV	RAYANNE	RAZI
RASTY	RAYANSH	RAZIA
RASUL	RAYCHEL	RAZIK
RATEEL	RAYCHELLE	RAZIKA
RATU	RAYDAN	RAZIN
RAUF	RAYDEN	RAZINA
RAUL	RAYDON	RAZNA
RAUMAAN	RAYE	RAZVAN

RAZWAN	REDHA	REGGIE-JOE
RAZWANA	REDLEY	REGGIE-LEE
RE	REDMOND	REGGIE-RAE
RE'KAI	REDON	REGGIE-RAY
REA	REDOUANE	REGGY
REACE	REDVERS	REGINA
READE	REDWAN	REGINAE
REAF	REE	REGINALD
REAGAN	REEAN	REGIS
REAGEN	REECE	REHA
REAGON	REECE-JUNIOR	REHAAN
REAH	REECO	REHAB
REAM	REED	REHAM
REAN	REEF	REHAN
REANA	REEFE	REHANA
REANN	REEGAN	REHANNA
REANNA	REEHA	REHANNAH
REANNAH	REEHAM	REHEEM
REANNAN	REEHAN	REHEMA
REANNE	REEKO	REHMA
REANNON	REEM	REHMAAN
REAVE	REEMA	REHMAN
REBA	REEMAS	REHMAT
REBBECA	REENA	REHNUMA
REBBECCA	REENIE	REHOBOTH
REBBEKAH	REES	REI
REBECA	REESA	REIA
REBECCA	REESE	REIAN
REBECCA-JADE	REESHA	REICE
REBECCA-LOUISE	REET	REID
REBECCA-MAY	REETAL	REIF
REBECCA-ROSE	REEVA	REIGAN
REBECCAH	REEVE	REIGEN
REBECKA	REEVES	REIGHAN
REBECKAH	REEYA	REIGN
REBEKA	REEYAH	REIKO
REBEKAH	REEYAN	REILEY
REBEKHA	REFAEL	REILLEY
REBEKKA	REFOEL	REILLY
REBEKKAH	REG	REILY
REBWAR	REGA	REINA
RECEP	REGAN	REINE
RECO	REGAN-LEE	REINIER
RED	REGEN	REINIS
REDA	REGGI	REION
REDAS	REGGIE	REIS
REDD	REGGIE-JAMES	REISA
REDFORD	REGGIE-JAY	REISE

REISEL
REISHA
REISS
REISY
REIVA
REIYA
REIZEL
REIZY
REJA
REJAN
REJOICE
REJUS
REJWAN
REJWANA
REKA
REKAI
REKAN
REKAR
REKHA
REM
REMA
REMAE
REMAI
REMAN
REMARI
REMARIO
REMARNI
REMAS
REMAY
REMAYA
REMAYAH
REMAZ
REME
REMEE
REMEL
REMELL
REMI
REMI-LEIGH
REMI-MAE
REMI-ROSE
REMIAH
REMIE
REMIEL
REMIGIUSZ
REMILEKUN
REMINGTON
REMIREZ
REMIYAH

REMMEL
REMMI
REMMIE
REMMY
REMO
REMUS
REMY
REMY-LEIGH
REMZI
REN
RENA
RENAD
RENAE
RENAEYAH
RENAI
RENAIYA
RENALDAS
RENALDO
RENAN
RENARS
RENAS
RENAT
RENATA
RENATO
RENAY
RENAYA
RENAYAH
RENAYE
RENDIJS
RENE
RENEA
RENEE
RENEECE
RENEL
RENELL
RENELLE
RENESH
RENESMAE
RENESMAI
RENESMAY
RENESME
RENESMEE
RENESMEE-JANE
RENEYA
RENEZMAE
RENEZMAI
RENGIN
RENI

RENIE
RENIECE
RENIS
RENITA
RENIYAH
RENLEY
RENLY
RENN
RENNA
RENNAE
RENNEL
RENNIE
RENNY
RENO
RENU
RENUKA
RENWA
RENZ
RENZO
REO
REON
RERELOLUWA
RESHA
RESHAM
RESHAUN
RESHMA
RESHMI
RESMA
RESUL
RETAAJ
RETAAL
RETAJ
RETAL
REUBAN
REUBEN
REUBEN-JAMES
REUBEN-LEE
REUBIN
REUBYN
REUEL
REUVEN
REVA
REVAH
REVAN
REVE
REWAN
REX
REXFORD

REXHEP	RHIANAN	RHYLEE
REXLEY	RHIANE	RHYLEIGH
REY	RHIANEDD	RHYLEY
REYA	RHIANN	RHYLIE
REYAAN	RHIANNA	RHYON
REYAANSH	RHIANNA-MAE	RHYS
REYAH	RHIANNAH	RHYS-JAMES
REYAN	RHIANNAN	RHYSE
REYANA	RHIANNE	RHYSS
REYANNE	RHIANNON	RHYTHM
REYANSH	RHIANON	RHYZ
REYES	RHIANWEN	RIA
REYHAN	RHIANYDD	RIA-MAY
REYHANA	RHIARNA	RIAAN
REYNA	RHIDIAN	RIAD
REYNARD	RHIEN	RIADEEP
REYNOLD	RHILEY	RIAH
REYO	RHION	RIAHANNA
REYON	RHITIK	RIAIN
REYYAN	RHIYA	RIAN
REZA	RHIYAN	RIANA
REZWAN	RHOAN	RIANAH
REZWANA	RHOANNE	RIANE
RHAIN	RHODA	RIANN
RHAYA	RHODES	RIANNA
RHEA	RHODRI	RIANNAH
RHEAGAN	RHOME	RIANNAN
RHEAN	RHONA	RIANNE
RHEANA	RHONAN	RIANNON
RHEANN	RHONDA	RIARNA
RHEANNA	RHONWEN	RIAZ
RHEANNAN	RHOSLYN	RIBQAH
RHEANNE	RHOSWEN	RICA
RHEANNON	RHOSYN	RICARDA
RHEECE	RHUBEN	RICARDAS
RHEGAN	RHUN	RICARDO
RHEIA	RHY	RICARDS
RHEMA	RHYA	RICCARDO
RHEO	RHYAN	RICCI
RHEON	RHYANA	RICCO
RHETT	RHYANN	RICH
RHEUBEN	RHYANNA	RICHA
RHEYA	RHYANNE	RICHARD
RHIA	RHYANNON	RICHARDO
RHIAD	RHYCE	RICHELLE
RHIAIN	RHYDER	RICHIE
RHIAN	RHYDIAN	RICHIE-LEE
RHIANA	RHYLAN	RICHMOND

RICHY
RICK
RICKARDO
RICKESH
RICKEY
RICKI
RICKIE
RICKY
RICKY-JUNIOR
RICKY-LEE
RICKYLEE
RICO
RICOH
RIDA
RIDAA
RIDAH
RIDAS
RIDDHI
RIDDICK
RIDHA
RIDHAAN
RIDHAM
RIDHI
RIDHIMA
RIDHWAAN
RIDHWAN
RIDLEY
RIDWAAN
RIDWAN
RIDWANA
RIDWANAH
RIECE
RIEGAN
RIELEY
RIELLA
RIELLE
RIELLY
RIELY
RIEN
RIFA
RIFAH
RIFAT
RIFKA
RIFKI
RIFKY
RIGA
RIGBY
RIHA

RIHAAM
RIHAAN
RIHAANA
RIHAB
RIHAM
RIHAN
RIHANA
RIHANAH
RIHANAT
RIHANN
RIHANNA
RIHANNA-MAI
RIHANNAH
RIHANNE
RIHANNON
RIHARDS
RIISE
RIJA
RIJJA
RIJUL
RIK
RIKA
RIKAI
RIKARDO
RIKAYA
RIKEN
RIKESH
RIKHIL
RIKI
RIKIN
RIKITA
RIKKI
RIKKY
RIKO
RIKU
RILAN
RILEE
RILEIGH
RILEY
RILEY-
RILEY-DEAN
RILEY-GEORGE
RILEY-J
RILEY-JACK
RILEY-JAE
RILEY-JAI
RILEY-JAMES
RILEY-JAY

RILEY-JOE
RILEY-JOHN
RILEY-LEE
RILEY-MAE
RILEY-MASON
RILEY-PAUL
RILEY-RAY
RILEY-ROSE
RILEY-SCOTT
RILEY-THOMAS
RILIND
RILLEY
RILWAN
RILY
RIM
RIMA
RIMAH
RIMAS
RIMI
RIMINI
RIMMEL
RIMON
RIMSHA
RIMSHAH
RINA
RINAAD
RINAD
RINAH
RINALDS
RINESA
RINGO
RINI
RINNAH
RINOA
RINOR
RIO
RIO-JAMES
RIOJA
RION
RIONA
RIORDAN
RIPA
RIPLEY
RIQUELME
RISA
RISAKO
RISH
RISHA

RISHAAN	RIVER-MAE	ROBBYN
RISHAB	RIVER-RAE	ROBEL
RISHABH	RIVER-ROSE	ROBEN
RISHAD	RIVERS	ROBERT
RISHAL	RIVIERA	ROBERT-JAMES
RISHAN	RIVKA	ROBERT-LEE
RISHANA	RIVKAH	ROBERTA
RISHANTH	RIVKY	ROBERTAS
RISHARN	RIYA	ROBERTO
RISHAV	RIYAAD	ROBERTS
RISHAY	RIYAADH	ROBI
RISHI	RIYAAN	ROBIN
RISHIK	RIYAAZ	ROBINA
RISHIKA	RIYAD	ROBINSON
RISHIKESH	RIYADH	ROBIUL
RISHIL	RIYADHUL	ROBLEH
RISHIT	RIYADUL	ROBSON
RISHITA	RIYAH	ROBY
RISHITHA	RIYAN	ROBYN
RISHON	RIYANA	ROBYN-LEIGH
RITA	RIYANNA	ROBYN-RAE
RITAJ	RIYANSH	ROBYN-ROSE
RITAL	RIYANSHI	ROBYNE
RITANYA	RIYAZ	ROBYNN
RITCHIE	RIYEN	ROBYNNE
RITESH	RIYON	ROC
RITHIK	RIYYAN	ROCCO
RITHIKA	RIZA	ROCCO-LEE
RITHISH	RIZWAAN	ROCH
RITHVIK	RIZWAN	ROCHAN
RITHWIK	RIZWANA	ROCHANA
RITI	RJ	ROCHE
RITIK	ROA	ROCHEL
RITIKA	ROAA	ROCHELLE
RITISHA	ROALD	ROCIO
RITU	ROAN	ROCK
RITVI	ROANNA	ROCKET
RITVIK	ROANNE	ROCKIE
RIVA	ROARK	ROCKO
RIVAAN	ROARKE	ROCKY
RIVAH	ROARY	ROCO
RIVALDO	ROB	ROD
RIVAN	ROBA	RODA
RIVEN	ROBAT	RODAINA
RIVER	ROBBERT	RODAS
RIVER-LEA	ROBBIE	RODDY
RIVER-LEE	ROBBIE-LEE	RODELA
RIVER-LEIGH	ROBBY	RODERICK

RODI	ROLANDO	ROMERO
RODIN	ROLF	ROMESA
RODINA	ROLLO	ROMESH
RODNEY	ROMA	ROMESSA
RODRIGO	ROMAAN	ROMEY
ROEL	ROMAANA	ROMI
ROEN	ROMAE	ROMIE
ROGAN	ROMAEO	ROMILLIE
ROGEN	ROMAHN	ROMILLY
ROGER	ROMAI	ROMILY
ROGUE	ROMAIN	ROMINA
ROHA	ROMAINE	ROMIR
ROHAAN	ROMAIO	ROMMEL
ROHAIL	ROMAISA	ROMOLA
ROHAM	ROMAL	ROMONE
ROHAN	ROMAN	ROMY
ROHANA	ROMAN-JAMES	RON
ROHANNA	ROMAN-LEE	RONA
ROHAT	ROMANA	RONAK
ROHEEL	ROMANE	RONALD
ROHEN	ROMANI	RONALDAS
ROHEY	ROMANIE	RONALDINHO
ROHID	ROMANII	RONALDO
ROHIL	ROMANN	RONAN
ROHIMA	ROMANO	RONAR
ROHIN	ROMANS	RONAV
ROHINA	ROMANY	RONAY
ROHINI	ROMANY-ROSE	RONDA
ROHIT	ROMAO	RONEL
ROHITH	ROMAR	RONELA
ROHN	ROMAREO	RONELL
ROI	ROMARI	RONI
ROISIN	ROMARIO	RONIA
ROJ	ROMARNI	RONICA
ROJA	ROMARNO	RONIE
ROJAN	ROMAYA	RONIK
ROJBIN	ROMAYNE	RONIKA
ROJDA	ROMAYSA	RONIN
ROJHAT	ROME	RONIQUE
ROJIN	ROMEE	RONIT
ROJUS	ROMEESA	RONJA
ROKAS	ROMEL	RONN
ROKAYA	ROMELL	RONNELL
ROKO	ROMELLE	RONNI
ROKSANA	ROMELLO	RONNIE
ROLAN	ROMELO	RONNIE-GEORGE
ROLAND	ROMEN	RONNIE-JAMES
ROLANDA	ROMEO	RONNIE-JAY

RONNIE-JUNIOR	ROSAMUND	ROSIE-
RONNIE-LEE	ROSANA	ROSIE-ANN
RONNIE-LEIGH	ROSANNA	ROSIE-ANNE
RONNIE-MAE	ROSANNAH	ROSIE-BELLE
RONNIE-MAY	ROSANNE	ROSIE-BETH
RONNIE-RAY	ROSARIA	ROSIE-GRACE
RONNIE-ROSE	ROSARIO	ROSIE-JANE
RONNY	ROSCO	ROSIE-LEA
RONON	ROSCOE	ROSIE-LEE
RONSON	ROSE	ROSIE-LEIGH
RONY	ROSE-ANN	ROSIE-LOU
RONYA	ROSE-ANNE	ROSIE-LOUISE
ROOHI	ROSE-ELLA	ROSIE-MAE
ROOMANA	ROSE-LEIGH	ROSIE-MAI
ROONEY	ROSE-MARIE	ROSIE-MARIE
ROOP	ROSEALIE	ROSIE-MAY
ROOS	ROSEANN	ROSIE-RAE
ROPAFADZO	ROSEANNA	ROSIELEIGH
ROQUE	ROSEANNAH	ROSINA
RORAN	ROSEANNE	ROSITA
ROREY	ROSELEEN	ROSKO
RORI	ROSELINE	ROSLYN
RORIE	ROSELLA	ROSS
RORY	ROSELLE	ROSSANA
RORY-JAMES	ROSELYN	ROSSCO
RORY-JAY	ROSEMARIE	ROSSELLA
ROSA	ROSEMARY	ROSSI
ROSA-BELLA	ROSEMIN	ROSSLYN
ROSA-LEA	ROSENA	ROSTAM
ROSA-LEIGH	ROSENWYN	ROSTISLAV
ROSABEL	ROSETTA	ROSY
ROSABELLA	ROSEY	ROUMAISSA
ROSABELLE	ROSH	ROURKE
ROSALEA	ROSHA	ROUX
ROSALEE	ROSHAAN	ROWAN
ROSALEEN	ROSHAN	ROWAN-JAMES
ROSALEIGH	ROSHANA	ROWANNE
ROSALIA	ROSHANAK	ROWAYDA
ROSALIE	ROSHANE	ROWDA
ROSALIN	ROSHANI	ROWEN
ROSALINA	ROSHAUN	ROWENA
ROSALIND	ROSHEEN	ROWENNA
ROSALINDA	ROSHELLE	ROWLAND
ROSALINE	ROSHEN	ROWLEY
ROSALITA	ROSHINI	ROXANA
ROSALYN	ROSHNI	ROXANE
ROSAMARIA	ROSI	ROXANN
ROSAMOND	ROSIE	ROXANNA

ROXANNE	RUBEN-JAMES	RUBY-MARIE
ROXI	RUBEN-LEE	RUBY-MAY
ROXI-LEIGH	RUBENA	RUBY-RAE
ROXIE	RUBENS	RUBY-ROSE
ROXXI	RUBI	RUBY-SUE
ROXY	RUBI-LEIGH	RUBY-SUMMER
ROXY-LEIGH	RUBI-MAE	RUBY-TUESDAY
ROY	RUBI-MAI	RUBY-VIOLET
ROYA	RUBI-ROSE	RUBYANN
ROYAL	RUBIA	RUBYANNE
ROYCE	RUBIE	RUBYLEE
ROYDON	RUBIE-LEIGH	RUBYLEIGH
ROYEM	RUBIE-LOUISE	RUBYMAY
ROYSTON	RUBIE-MAE	RUBYN
ROZ	RUBIE-MAI	RUBYROSE
ROZA	RUBIE-MAY	RUCHA
ROZALIA	RUBIE-ROSE	RUCHAMA
ROZAN	RUBIN	RUCHEL
ROZANA	RUBINA	RUCHI
ROZE	RUBINDER	RUCHIKA
ROZEENA	RUBIO	RUDAINA
ROZELIN	RUBY	RUDEY
ROZERIN	RUBY-	RUDHRA
ROZH	RUBY-ANN	RUDI
ROZI	RUBY-ANNA	RUDIE
ROZIE	RUBY-ANNE	RUDINA
ROZINA	RUBY-BLU	RUDO
ROZITA	RUBY-ELLA	RUDOLF
ROZY	RUBY-ELLEN	RUDOLPH
RRON	RUBY-FAITH	RUDR
RUA	RUBY-GRACE	RUDRA
RUADHAN	RUBY-JADE	RUDRAKSH
RUAIDHRI	RUBY-JAI	RUDRANSH
RUAIRI	RUBY-JANE	RUDWAN
RUAIRIDH	RUBY-JAYNE	RUDY
RUAN	RUBY-JEAN	RUDYARD
RUARAIDH	RUBY-JO	RUE
RUARI	RUBY-JOY	RUEBAN
RUARIDH	RUBY-JUNE	RUEBEN
RUBA	RUBY-LEA	RUEBEN-JAMES
RUBAAB	RUBY-LEE	RUEDI
RUBAB	RUBY-LEI	RUEL
RUBAN	RUBY-LEIGH	RUELLE
RUBANI	RUBY-LILLY	RUFAEL
RUBEE	RUBY-LOU	RUFAIDA
RUBEENA	RUBY-LOUISE	RUFAIDAH
RUBEL	RUBY-MAE	RUFARO
RUBEN	RUBY-MAI	RUFAYDAH

RUFUS	RUMAYSAA	RUSLANA
RUGILE	RUMAYSAH	RUSLANS
RUHAAN	RUMBIDZAI	RUSNE
RUHAB	RUMEISA	RUSSEL
RUHAL	RUMEL	RUSSELL
RUHAMA	RUMENA	RUSSELL-JAMES
RUHAN	RUMER	RUSTAM
RUHANI	RUMESA	RUSTY
RUHE	RUMESSA	RUT
RUHEE	RUMEYSA	RUTA
RUHEL	RUMI	RUTENDO
RUHENA	RUMINA	RUTH
RUHI	RUMMAN	RUTHIE
RUHIKA	RUMMANAH	RUTHVIK
RUHINA	RUMSHA	RUTVI
RUHMA	RUNA	RUTVIK
RUHUL	RUNAKO	RUVARASHE
RUI	RUNE	RUVIMBO
RUJINA	RUO	RUWAIDA
RUKAIYA	RUOXI	RUWAIDAH
RUKAIYAH	RUPA	RUWAN
RUKAYA	RUPALI	RUWAYDA
RUKAYAH	RUPEN	RUWAYDAH
RUKAYAT	RUPERT	RUWEYDA
RUKAYYA	RUPINDER	RUYA
RUKAYYAH	RUQAIYA	RUZENA
RUKEN	RUQAIYAH	RUZGAR
RUKHSAAR	RUQAIYYA	RUZINA
RUKHSANA	RUQAIYYAH	RWAN
RUKHSAR	RUQAYA	RY
RUKIA	RUQAYAH	RYA
RUKIYA	RUQAYYA	RYAAN
RUKIYE	RUQAYYAH	RYAD
RUKSAAR	RUQIA	RYAH
RUKSANA	RUQIYA	RYAN
RUKSAR	RUQIYAH	RYAN-JAMES
RUKSHANA	RUQQAYA	RYAN-JUNIOR
RUMA	RUQQAYAH	RYAN-LEE
RUMAAN	RUSHAN	RYANDEEP
RUMAANA	RUSHANE	RYANLEE
RUMAANAH	RUSHAUN	RYANN
RUMAISA	RUSHAWN	RYANNA
RUMAISAH	RUSHDA	RYANNE
RUMAITHAH	RUSHI	RYANVEER
RUMAN	RUSHIKA	RYDAL
RUMANA	RUSHIL	RYDAN
RUMANAH	RUSHNA	RYDEN
RUMAYSA	RUSLAN	RYDER

RYDER-JAMES
RYE
RYELL
RYEN
RYHAN
RYHANA
RYHANNA
RYHS
RYKER
RYLA
RYLAN
RYLAND
RYLE
RYLEA
RYLEE
RYLEE-JAMES
RYLEE-JAY
RYLEI
RYLEIGH
RYLEIGH-MAE
RYLEN
RYLEY
RYLEY-JAMES
RYLEY-JAY
RYLI
RYLIE
RYLY
RYM
RYNAD
RYO
RYOMA
RYON
RYOSUKE
RYOTA
RYSZARD
RYU
RYVER
RYYAN

S

S	SAANYA	SABILA
SA'AD	SAAQIB	SABIN
SAABIR	SAARA	SABINA
SAABIRIN	SAARAA	SABINE
SAACHI	SAARAH	SABIQ
SAAD	SAARIM	SABIR
SAADA	SAARIYAH	SABIRA
SAADI	SAARRAH	SABIRAH
SAADIA	SAARTH	SABIRIIN
SAADIAH	SAATHANA	SABIRIN
SAADIQ	SAATHVIK	SABIYA
SAADIYA	SAATVIK	SABIYAH
SAADIYAH	SAAVAN	SABOOR
SAAGAR	SAAVI	SABRA
SAAHIBAH	SAAYA	SABREEN
SAAHIL	SABA	SABREENA
SAAHIR	SABAA	SABRENA
SAAHIRAH	SABAAH	SABRI
SAAID	SABAH	SABRIIN
SAAIM	SABAHAT	SABRIN
SAAIMA	SABANA	SABRINA
SAAIMAH	SABARIN	SABRINE
SAAIRAH	SABASTIAN	SABRIYA
SAAJAN	SABBA	SABRIYAH
SAAJID	SABBAH	SACARIO
SAAJIDAH	SABBIR	SACHA
SAALEH	SABEEH	SACHELLE
SAALEHA	SABEEHA	SACHI
SAALIH	SABEEHAH	SACHIN
SAALIHA	SABEEKA	SACHIT
SAALIHAH	SABEEL	SACHITH
SAAM	SABEELA	SACHLEEN
SAAMI	SABEEN	SACHPREET
SAAMIA	SABEENA	SADA
SAAMIR	SABEEQA	SADAF
SAAMIYA	SABEER	SADAN
SAAMIYAH	SABEERA	SADAQ
SAAN	SABELLA	SADAQAT
SAANA	SABENA	SADDIQ
SAANIA	SABER	SADE
SAANIYA	SABERA	SADEED
SAANIYAH	SABHA	SADEEL
SAANVI	SABIA	SADEEM
SAANVIKA	SABIAH	SADEKA
	SABIAN	SADHANA
	SABIH	SADHBH
	SABIHA	SADHIA
	SABIHAH	SADIA

SADIAH	SAFFIE	SAHAB
SADIE	SAFFINA	SAHAD
SADIE-GRACE	SAFFIR	SAHAIR
SADIE-LEIGH	SAFFIRA	SAHAJ
SADIE-MAE	SAFFIRE	SAHAJDEEP
SADIE-MAY	SAFFIYA	SAHAL
SADIE-RAE	SAFFIYAH	SAHAM
SADIE-ROSE	SAFFIYYAH	SAHAN
SADIK	SAFFRON	SAHANA
SADIKA	SAFHA	SAHAND
SADIKUR	SAFI	SAHAR
SADIQ	SAFIA	SAHARA
SADIQA	SAFIAH	SAHARAH
SADIQAH	SAFIAN	SAHARSH
SADIQUL	SAFIATOU	SAHAS
SADIQUR	SAFIN	SAHASRA
SADIYA	SAFINA	SAHD
SADIYAH	SAFIRA	SAHDIA
SADIYYA	SAFIRE	SAHEB
SADUF	SAFIULLAH	SAHEEL
SADYA	SAFIYA	SAHEIM
SAE	SAFIYAH	SAHEJ
SAED	SAFIYAN	SAHEL
SAEED	SAFIYE	SAHER
SAEEDA	SAFIYO	SAHERA
SAEEDAH	SAFIYYA	SAHIB
SAEEM	SAFIYYAH	SAHIBA
SAEMA	SAFOORA	SAHIBAH
SAESHA	SAFOORAH	SAHIBDEEP
SAFA	SAFRAZ	SAHIBJEET
SAFAA	SAFREEN	SAHIBJOT
SAFAAH	SAFRON	SAHIBPREET
SAFAH	SAFURA	SAHIBVEER
SAFAL	SAFURAH	SAHIBVIR
SAFANA	SAFWA	SAHIBZADA
SAFARI	SAFWAAN	SAHID
SAFEENA	SAFWAN	SAHIDA
SAFEENAH	SAFWANA	SAHIJ
SAFEER	SAFYA	SAHIL
SAFEERA	SAFYAAN	SAHILL
SAFEERAH	SAFYAN	SAHIM
SAFEEYA	SAGA	SAHIMA
SAFEEYAH	SAGAL	SAHIN
SAFFA	SAGANA	SAHIR
SAFFAH	SAGAR	SAHIRA
SAFFANAH	SAGE	SAHL
SAFFI	SAHA	SAHLA
SAFFIA	SAHAANA	SAHR

SAHRA	SAIYAM	SALAHUDIN
SAHRISH	SAIYAN	SALAM
SAHUR	SAIYARA	SALAR
SAI	SAIYEDA	SALEEHA
SAIBA	SAJA	SALEEM
SAIBAH	SAJAD	SALEEMA
SAID	SAJAL	SALEEMAH
SAIDA	SAJAN	SALEENA
SAIDAH	SAJANA	SALEH
SAIDOU	SAJDA	SALEHA
SAIED	SAJDAH	SALEHAH
SAIEM	SAJED	SALEISHA
SAIF	SAJEDA	SALEM
SAIF-ALI	SAJEEL	SALEMA
SAIF-ULLAH	SAJEEV	SALENA
SAIFA	SAJID	SALHA
SAIFAAN	SAJIDA	SALI
SAIFALI	SAJIDAH	SALIA
SAIFAN	SAJIDUR	SALIAH
SAIFUDDIN	SAJITH	SALIEU
SAIFUL	SAJJAD	SALIH
SAIFULLAH	SAJJAN	SALIHA
SAIFUR	SAJMON	SALIHAH
SAIGE	SAJNI	SALIK
SAIHAAN	SAKARA	SALIM
SAIHAJ	SAKARIA	SALIMA
SAIHAJLEEN	SAKARIYA	SALIMAH
SAIHAN	SAKARIYE	SALIMATOU
SAIHOU	SAKEENA	SALINA
SAIKA	SAKEENAH	SALLAH
SAIKOU	SAKETH	SALLIE
SAILOR	SAKI	SALLY
SAIM	SAKIB	SALLY-ANN
SAIMA	SAKINA	SALLY-ANNE
SAIMAH	SAKINAH	SALLYANN
SAIMON	SAKO	SALMA
SAIMONAS	SAKSHAM	SALMAA
SAINA	SAKSHI	SALMAAN
SAINABOU	SAKURA	SALMAH
SAINT	SALAAH	SALMAN
SAINTHAVI	SALAAR	SALMO
SAIQA	SALADIN	SALOME
SAIRA	SALAH	SALOMEA
SAIRAH	SALAH-UDDIN	SALOMEIA
SAIRISH	SALAHADIN	SALOMON
SAISH	SALAHUDDEEN	SALONI
SAISHA	SALAHUDDIN	SALSABEEL
SAIYA	SALAHUDEEN	SALSABIL

SALUM	SAMEED	SAMIULLAH
SALVADOR	SAMEEHA	SAMIUR
SALVATORE	SAMEEKSHA	SAMIYA
SALWA	SAMEEL	SAMIYAH
SAM	SAMEEM	SAMM
SAMA	SAMEEN	SAMMA
SAMAA	SAMEENA	SAMMAN
SAMAAD	SAMEENAH	SAMMAR
SAMAAH	SAMEER	SAMMER
SAMAD	SAMEERA	SAMMI
SAMAH	SAMEERAH	SAMMI-JO
SAMAHER	SAMEET	SAMMIA
SAMAIRA	SAMEEYA	SAMMIE
SAMAIYA	SAMEH	SAMMIE-JO
SAMAN	SAMENA	SAMMUEL
SAMANA	SAMER	SAMMY
SAMANDA	SAMERA	SAMMY-JO
SAMANTA	SAMERAH	SAMMY-LEE
SAMANTHA	SAMESH	SAMMYA
SAMANTHA-JANE	SAMET	SAMMYJO
SAMANTHA-JAYNE	SAMEUL	SAMPREET
SAMANTHA-JO	SAMEYA	SAMPSON
SAMANTHA-LOUISE	SAMHA	SAMRA
SAMANVI	SAMHITA	SAMRAAJ
SAMANYU	SAMHITHA	SAMRAAT
SAMAR	SAMI	SAMRAH
SAMARA	SAMI-UL	SAMRAJ
SAMARAH	SAMI-ULLAH	SAMRAN
SAMARBIR	SAMIA	SAMRAT
SAMARDEEP	SAMIAH	SAMRATH
SAMARIA	SAMIAT	SAMRAWIT
SAMARITEANCA	SAMIE	SAMREEN
SAMARJOT	SAMIH	SAMREET
SAMARPREET	SAMIHA	SAMRIDDHI
SAMARRA	SAMIHAH	SAMRIDHI
SAMARTH	SAMIIRA	SAMSAM
SAMARVEER	SAMIK	SAMSON
SAMARVIR	SAMIKA	SAMUAL
SAMATAR	SAMIKSHA	SAMUEL
SAMAY	SAMIM	SAMUEL-JAMES
SAMAYA	SAMIN	SAMUELA
SAMBA	SAMINA	SAMUELE
SAMBHAV	SAMIP	SAMUELL
SAMBOR	SAMIR	SAMUELLA
SAMED	SAMIRA	SAMUIL
SAMEE	SAMIRAH	SAMVEER
SAMEEA	SAMIT	SAMVIR
SAMEEAH	SAMIUL	SAMY

SAMYA
SAMYAN
SAMYAR
SAMYOG
SAMYRA
SAMYUKTHA
SAN
SANA
SANAA
SANAAH
SANAD
SANAH
SANAIYA
SANAM
SANAN
SANAV
SANAYA
SANAYAH
SANAZ
SANCHA
SANCHEZ
SANCHI
SANCHIA
SANCHIT
SANCHO
SANCIA
SANDEEP
SANDER
SANDHYA
SANDI
SANDIE
SANDILE
SANDIP
SANDIS
SANDOR
SANDRA
SANDRO
SANDY
SANEELA
SANEESH
SANEHA
SANEL
SANELA
SANEM
SANG
SANGAVI
SANGEETA
SANHA

SANI
SANIA
SANIAH
SANIHA
SANIJA
SANIKA
SANIL
SANITA
SANIYA
SANIYAH
SANIYYA
SANIYYAH
SANJANA
SANJAY
SANJEEDA
SANJEET
SANJEEV
SANJEEVAN
SANJIDA
SANJIDAH
SANJIT
SANJITH
SANJIV
SANJNA
SANJOG
SANJU
SANKALP
SANKAVI
SANNA
SANNAH
SANNE
SANSA
SANSAR
SANSKRITI
SANTA
SANTAE
SANTANA
SANTANNA
SANTHIYA
SANTHOSH
SANTHYA
SANTI
SANTIAGO
SANTINA
SANTINO
SANTO
SANTOS
SANTOSH

SANULI
SANUSI
SANUTHI
SANVEER
SANVI
SANVIKA
SANVIR
SANYA
SANYAH
SAOIRSE
SAONA
SAOOD
SAORLAITH
SAPHIA
SAPHINA
SAPHIR
SAPHIRA
SAPHIRE
SAPHIYA
SAPHORA
SAPHRON
SAPHYRE
SAPNA
SAPPHIRA
SAPPHIRE
SAPPHIRE-MARIE
SAPPHIRE-ROSE
SAQAB
SAQIB
SAQLAIN
SARA
SARA-JANE
SARA-JAYNE
SARA-LOUISE
SARAA
SARACEN
SARAFINA
SARAH
SARAH-
SARAH-ANN
SARAH-ANNE
SARAH-BETH
SARAH-JANE
SARAH-JAYNE
SARAH-LOU
SARAH-LOUISE
SARAH-MARIE
SARAH-MAY

SARAH-ROSE
SARAHJANE
SARAHLOUISE
SARAI
SARAIYA
SARAIYAH
SARAM
SARAN
SARANG
SARANNE
SARANYA
SARAVANAN
SARAYA
SARAYAH
SARAYU
SARBJEET
SARBJIT
SARDAR
SARE
SAREEN
SAREENA
SAREM
SARENA
SARENNA
SAREYA
SARFARAZ
SARFRAZ
SARGUN
SARI
SARIA
SARIAH
SARIKA
SARIM
SARINA
SARINAH
SARISH
SARISHA
SARITA
SARIYA
SARIYAH
SARJAN
SARJUN
SARLOTA
SARLOTE
SARMAD
SARO
SARON
SAROOP

SAROSH
SARP
SARRA
SARRAH
SARRINA
SARRINAH
SARTAAJ
SARTAJ
SARTHAK
SARUJAN
SARUNAS
SARVAN
SARVESH
SARWA
SARWAR
SARYA
SASAN
SASCHA
SASHA
SASHA-LOUISE
SASHA-MAE
SASHI
SASHINI
SASHKA
SASHVIN
SASKA
SASKIA
SASKYA
SASSI
SASWIN
SATBIR
SATHANA
SATHUSAN
SATHVIK
SATHVIKA
SATINDER
SATINE
SATISH
SATNAM
SATPAL
SATPREET
SATSUKI
SATVEER
SATVIK
SATVIR
SATWINDER
SATYA
SATYAM

SAUD
SAUDA
SAUDAH
SAUGAT
SAUL
SAULE
SAUMYA
SAURAV
SAVA
SAVAIN
SAVAIRA
SAVAN
SAVANA
SAVANAGH
SAVANAH
SAVANHA
SAVANNA
SAVANNA-ROSE
SAVANNAH
SAVANNAH-GRACE
SAVANNAH-LEIGH
SAVANNAH-LOUISE
SAVANNAH-MAE
SAVANNAH-MAI
SAVANNAH-RAE
SAVANNAH-ROSE
SAVARNA
SAVAS
SAVERA
SAVERAH
SAVIA
SAVINA
SAVIO
SAVIOUR
SAVIR
SAVIRA
SAVITA
SAVO
SAVRAAJ
SAVRAJ
SAVREEN
SAVVA
SAVVAS
SAVYA
SAWAIRA
SAWAN
SAWDA
SAWDAH

SAWERA	SCARLETT-ANN	SEDA
SAWSAN	SCARLETT-ANNE	SEDANUR
SAWYER	SCARLETT-GRACE	SEDAT
SAXON	SCARLETT-JADE	SEDEF
SAYA	SCARLETT-JANE	SEDONA
SAYAAM	SCARLETT-LEA	SEDRA
SAYAM	SCARLETT-LEIGH	SEELEY
SAYAN	SCARLETT-LILLY	SEEMA
SAYANA	SCARLETT-LILY	SEEMAB
SAYDA	SCARLETT-LOUISE	SEENA
SAYDEE	SCARLETT-MAE	SEERAT
SAYED	SCARLETT-MAI	SEERIT
SAYEDA	SCARLETT-MARIE	SEETA
SAYEED	SCARLETT-MAY	SEETAL
SAYEEDA	SCARLETT-OLIVIA	SEFA
SAYEF	SCARLETT-RAE	SEFORA
SAYEM	SCARLETT-ROSE	SEGUN
SAYEMA	SCARLETTE	SEHAJ
SAYER	SCARLETTE-ROSE	SEHAJDEEP
SAYESHA	SCARLOTT	SEHAJPREET
SAYF	SCARLOTTE	SEHAJVEER
SAYFUL	SCHYLER	SEHAM
SAYFULLAH	SCOT	SEHAR
SAYHAAN	SCOTT	SEHEJ
SAYHAN	SCOTT-LEE	SEHER
SAYID	SCOTTY	SEHJ
SAYIDA	SCOUT	SEHR
SAYIM	SE	SEHREEN
SAYLA	SEAMAS	SEHRISH
SAYLOR	SEAMUS	SEIF
SAYMA	SEAN	SEIJI
SAYMON	SEAN-JUNIOR	SEIM
SAYNAB	SEAN-PAUL	SEIRIAN
SAYON	SEANA	SEJAL
SAYRA	SEANAGH	SEKINAT
SAYSHA	SEANN	SEKOU
SAYURI	SEANNA	SELA
SAYYAM	SEANPAUL	SELAH
SAYYED	SEB	SELAM
SAYYEDA	SEBA	SELASE
SAYYID	SEBASTIAAN	SELBY
SAYYIDA	SEBASTIAN	SELCUK
SAYYIDAH	SEBASTIANAS	SELDA
SCARLA	SEBASTIANO	SELEN
SCARLET	SEBASTIANS	SELENA
SCARLET-LOUISE	SEBASTIAO	SELENE
SCARLET-ROSE	SEBASTIEN	SELIHOM
SCARLETT	SEBASTION	SELIKEM

SELIM	SERAI	SERRA
SELIN	SERAIAH	SERREN
SELINA	SERAJ	SERYN
SELINAY	SERAN	SETAISH
SELINE	SERAPHIM	SETARA
SELMA	SERAPHINA	SETAREH
SELORM	SERAPHINE	SETAYESH
SELVI	SERAY	SETH
SELWYN	SERAYA	SETHAN
SEM	SERAYAH	SETHIKA
SEMA	SERCAN	SETHUKI
SEMANUR	SERDAR	SEUMAS
SEMHAR	SEREEN	SEUNG
SEMIH	SEREENA	SEVA
SEMILORE	SEREF	SEVAK
SEMIRA	SEREL	SEVAL
SEMRA	SEREN	SEVAN
SEN	SEREN-GRACE	SEVCAN
SENA	SEREN-HAF	SEVDA
SENADA	SEREN-LOUISE	SEVE
SENAN	SEREN-RAE	SEVEN
SENARA	SEREN-ROSE	SEVERIANO
SENAY	SERENA	SEVERINE
SENEL	SERENAH	SEVERYN
SENEM	SERENDIPITY	SEVGI
SENER	SERENE	SEVIL
SENIZ	SERENITY	SEVILAY
SENNA	SERENNA	SEVIM
SENNAN	SEREYA	SEVIN
SENNEN	SERGE	SEVVAL
SENON	SERGEI	SEWA
SENTHOORAN	SERGEN	SEWERYN
SENUKA	SERGEY	SEYAM
SENULI	SERGIO	SEYAR
SENYO	SERGIU	SEYDA
SEO	SERGIUSZ	SEYED
SEON	SERHAN	SEYEDEH
SEONA	SERHAT	SEYIT
SEONAID	SERI	SEYMA
SEPEHR	SERIAH	SEYMOUR
SEPH	SERIFE	SEYNABOU
SEPHORA	SERIGNE	SEYON
SEQUOIA	SERIN	SEYSHA
SERA	SERINA	SEZEN
SERAFIM	SERINE	SEZER
SERAFIN	SERISH	SEZGIN
SERAFINA	SERKAN	SHA
SERAH	SERPIL	SHAAHID

SHAAKIR	SHAFIN	SHAHMIR
SHAAKIRAH	SHAFIQ	SHAHNAWAZ
SHAAM	SHAFIUL	SHAHNAZ
SHAAN	SHAFIYA	SHAHNOOR
SHAANA	SHAFQAT	SHAHRAM
SHAANDEEP	SHAGANA	SHAHREEN
SHAANI	SHAGUFTA	SHAHRIA
SHAANPREET	SHAH	SHAHRIAR
SHAANTI	SHAHAAB	SHAHRIN
SHAANVI	SHAHAAN	SHAHRIYAR
SHAARAV	SHAHAB	SHAHROZ
SHABAAN	SHAHAD	SHAHRUKH
SHABAAZ	SHAHADOT	SHAHRYAR
SHABAN	SHAHAN	SHAHVEZ
SHABANA	SHAHANA	SHAHWAIZ
SHABAZ	SHAHANAZ	SHAHYAAN
SHABAZZ	SHAHARA	SHAHYAN
SHABBIR	SHAHARIAR	SHAHZAD
SHABIHA	SHAHARYAR	SHAHZADA
SHABINA	SHAHBAAZ	SHAHZADI
SHABIR	SHAHBAZ	SHAHZAIB
SHABNAM	SHAHD	SHAHZAIN
SHABNAZ	SHAHED	SHAHZEB
SHABNUM	SHAHEDA	SHAI
SHAD	SHAHEED	SHAIANNE
SHADA	SHAHEEM	SHAID
SHADAB	SHAHEEN	SHAIDA
SHADAE	SHAHEENA	SHAIDEN
SHADDAI	SHAHEER	SHAIDON
SHADE	SHAHEIM	SHAIK
SHADEN	SHAHEL	SHAIKH
SHADI	SHAHENA	SHAIKHA
SHADIA	SHAHID	SHAILA
SHADIYA	SHAHIDA	SHAILAH
SHADMAN	SHAHIDUL	SHAILAN
SHADRACH	SHAHIDUR	SHAILEE
SHADY	SHAHIL	SHAILEN
SHAE	SHAHIMA	SHAILENE
SHAEDON	SHAHIN	SHAILI
SHAELA	SHAHINA	SHAIMA
SHAELEIGH	SHAHINUR	SHAIMAA
SHAFA	SHAHIR	SHAIN
SHAFAQ	SHAHIRA	SHAINA
SHAFAY	SHAHIRAH	SHAINDY
SHAFAYAT	SHAHISTA	SHAINE
SHAFEE	SHAHJAHAN	SHAIRA
SHAFI	SHAHLA	SHAISTA
SHAFIA	SHAHMEER	SHAIVI

SHAIYA	SHALIN	SHAMREZ
SHAIYAN	SHALINA	SHAMS
SHAIZA	SHALINI	SHAMSA
SHAJAN	SHALIYAH	SHAMSHER
SHAJEDA	SHALOM	SHAMSUL
SHAJIDA	SHALONA	SHAMUS
SHAKA	SHAM	SHAMYA
SHAKAI	SHAMA	SHAMYLA
SHAKANA	SHAMAILA	SHAN
SHAKAR	SHAMAL	SHANA
SHAKARA	SHAMAR	SHANAAYA
SHAKAYLA	SHAMARA	SHANADE
SHAKEAL	SHAMARI	SHANAE
SHAKEEB	SHAMAS	SHANAI
SHAKEEL	SHAMAYA	SHANAIA
SHAKEELA	SHAMEEL	SHANAIYA
SHAKEELAH	SHAMEELA	SHANAIYAH
SHAKEEM	SHAMEELAH	SHANAN
SHAKEERA	SHAMEEM	SHANARA
SHAKEIL	SHAMEENA	SHANAY
SHAKEIRA	SHAMEER	SHANAYA
SHAKELA	SHAMEKA	SHANAYAH
SHAKERA	SHAMEL	SHANAYE
SHAKIA	SHAMELIA	SHANAZ
SHAKIB	SHAMEN	SHANE
SHAKIEL	SHAMIA	SHANE-JUNIOR
SHAKIERA	SHAMIAH	SHANEA
SHAKIL	SHAMIKA	SHANECE
SHAKILA	SHAMIL	SHANEE
SHAKINA	SHAMILA	SHANEECE
SHAKIR	SHAMILAH	SHANEEKA
SHAKIRA	SHAMILLA	SHANEEL
SHAKIRA-LEE	SHAMIM	SHANEEN
SHAKIRAH	SHAMIMA	SHANEI
SHAKIYA	SHAMIN	SHANEICE
SHAKIYAH	SHAMINA	SHANEIL
SHAKTHI	SHAMIR	SHANEKA
SHAKTI	SHAMIRA	SHANEL
SHAKUR	SHAMIRAH	SHANELA
SHAKYE	SHAMISO	SHANELL
SHAKYRA	SHAMITA	SHANELLA
SHALA	SHAMIYA	SHANELLE
SHALAMAR	SHAMLA	SHANEQUA
SHALEEN	SHAMMAH	SHANESE
SHALEIGH	SHAMMAI	SHANESSA
SHALEN	SHAMMAS	SHANETTE
SHALEY	SHAMOYA	SHANEY
SHALIKA	SHAMRAIZ	SHANEYA

SHANEZ
SHANG
SHANI
SHANIA
SHANIAH
SHANICE
SHANIE
SHANIECE
SHANII
SHANIKA
SHANIL
SHANINE
SHANIQUA
SHANIQUE
SHANISE
SHANISHA
SHANITA
SHANIYA
SHANIYAH
SHANJIDA
SHANKAR
SHANLEIGH
SHANLEY
SHANNA
SHANNAE
SHANNAGH
SHANNAH
SHANNAI
SHANNAN
SHANNARA
SHANNAY
SHANNEL
SHANNELL
SHANNELLE
SHANNEN
SHANNI
SHANNIA
SHANNICE
SHANNIE
SHANNON
SHANNON-
SHANNON-LEE
SHANNON-LEIGH
SHANNON-LOUISE
SHANNON-MARIE
SHANNON-PAIGE
SHANNYN
SHANON
SHANTA
SHANTAE
SHANTAI
SHANTANA
SHANTAY
SHANTAYA
SHANTE
SHANTEL
SHANTELL
SHANTELLE
SHANTI
SHANTIA
SHANUM
SHANVI
SHANYA
SHANYAH
SHANYCE
SHANZA
SHANZAY
SHANZE
SHANZEY
SHAPLA
SHAQUAN
SHAQUANA
SHAQUIEL
SHAQUIELLE
SHAQUIL
SHAQUILE
SHAQUILL
SHAQUILLA
SHAQUILLE
SHARA
SHARAD
SHARAE
SHARAF
SHARAI
SHARAINE
SHARAN
SHARANDEEP
SHARANJEET
SHARANJIT
SHARANYA
SHARAYA
SHARAZ
SHARDAE
SHARDAI
SHARDAY
SHARDONAY
SHARDONNAY
SHAREE
SHAREEF
SHAREEFAH
SHAREEN
SHARELLE
SHARI
SHARIA
SHARIAH
SHARICE
SHARIF
SHARIFA
SHARIFAH
SHARIFF
SHARIKA
SHARINA
SHARIQ
SHARIQA
SHARISSE
SHARIYAH
SHARJEEL
SHARLA
SHARLEE
SHARLEEN
SHARLEEZ
SHARLENE
SHARLIE
SHARLOTTE
SHARLYN
SHARMA
SHARMAINE
SHARMAKE
SHARMARKE
SHARMEEN
SHARMEL
SHARMILA
SHARMIN
SHARMINA
SHARMINE
SHARN
SHARNA
SHARNAE
SHARNAH
SHARNAI
SHARNAY
SHARNE
SHARNEE
SHARNELL

SHARNELLE	SHAWANA	SHAZAIB
SHARNEY	SHAWN	SHAZAIN
SHARNI	SHAWNA	SHAZAN
SHARNIA	SHAWNEE	SHAZANA
SHARNIE	SHAWNIE	SHAZEB
SHARNNA	SHAWNNA	SHAZEDA
SHARNTAY	SHAY	SHAZIA
SHARON	SHAYA	SHAZIB
SHARONA	SHAYAAN	SHAZIDA
SHARONDEEP	SHAYAH	SHAZIL
SHARONJEET	SHAYAN	SHAZMA
SHARONJIT	SHAYANA	SHAZMEEN
SHAROZ	SHAYANN	SHAZMIN
SHARUJAN	SHAYANNA	SHAZNA
SHARUKESH	SHAYANNE	SHAZNAY
SHARUN	SHAYDA	SHAZNEY
SHARUSAN	SHAYDEN	SHEA
SHARVIL	SHAYDN	SHEAMUS
SHARVIN	SHAYDON	SHEANI
SHARWIN	SHAYE	SHEBA
SHASHANK	SHAYEN	SHEEHAN
SHASHWAT	SHAYLA	SHEEMA
SHASMEEN	SHAYLA-LOUISE	SHEENA
SHATHA	SHAYLA-MAE	SHEERAN
SHAUL	SHAYLA-MAI	SHEEREEN
SHAUN	SHAYLA-MAY	SHEETAL
SHAUNA	SHAYLA-RAE	SHEEZA
SHAUNA-LEA	SHAYLAH	SHEFALI
SHAUNA-LEIGH	SHAYLAN	SHEHAB
SHAUNA-MARIE	SHAYLEA	SHEHBAZ
SHAUNAGH	SHAYLEE	SHEHNAZ
SHAUNAH	SHAYLEI	SHEHREEN
SHAUNAK	SHAYLEIGH	SHEHROZ
SHAUNEE	SHAYLEN	SHEHROZE
SHAUNEY	SHAYLEY	SHEHRYAR
SHAUNI	SHAYLON	SHEHZAD
SHAUNIE	SHAYMA	SHEHZADI
SHAUNNA	SHAYMAA	SHEIK
SHAUNNAH	SHAYMUS	SHEIKA
SHAUNPAUL	SHAYNA	SHEIKH
SHAUNTAE	SHAYNE	SHEIKHA
SHAUNTELLE	SHAYNI	SHEIKHAH
SHAUNY	SHAYNIE	SHEIL
SHAURYA	SHAYON	SHEILA
SHAVON	SHAYYAN	SHEIMA
SHAVONNE	SHAZA	SHEINA
SHAW	SHAZAAD	SHEINDEL
SHAWAIZ	SHAZAD	SHEINDY

SHEK
SHEKERA
SHEKH
SHEKHINAH
SHEKINA
SHEKINAH
SHEKIRA
SHEKU
SHELAH
SHELAN
SHELBEY
SHELBI
SHELBIE
SHELBY
SHELBY-LEA
SHELBY-LEIGH
SHELBY-LOUISE
SHELBY-ROSE
SHELDON
SHELINA
SHELLBIE
SHELLBY
SHELLEY
SHELLIE
SHELLY
SHELTON
SHEM
SHEMA
SHEMAIAH
SHEMAR
SHEMIAH
SHEN
SHENA
SHENADE
SHENAE
SHENAI
SHENALI
SHENAY
SHENAYA
SHENAZ
SHENEECE
SHENEL
SHENELL
SHENELLE
SHENG
SHENICE
SHENIECE
SHENIKA

SHENIQUA
SHENISE
SHENIYA
SHENIZ
SHENNAI
SHEPHERD
SHER
SHERAE
SHERALEE
SHERALYN
SHERAZ
SHEREE
SHEREECE
SHEREEN
SHEREENA
SHERELLE
SHERENA
SHERENE
SHERI
SHERICA
SHERICE
SHERIDAN
SHERIDEN
SHERIE
SHERIECE
SHERIF
SHERIFAT
SHERIFF
SHERIKA
SHERILYN
SHERIN
SHERINA
SHERINE
SHERISE
SHERISH
SHERISSE
SHERLOCK
SHERLYN
SHERNICE
SHERONA
SHERRELL
SHERRI
SHERRIDAN
SHERRIE
SHERRY
SHERVIN
SHERWIN
SHERYAAR

SHERYAR
SHERYL
SHEVA
SHEVANI
SHEVAUN
SHEVONNE
SHEY
SHEYA
SHEYLA
SHEZA
SHEZAD
SHI
SHIA
SHIALA
SHIAN
SHIANA
SHIANE
SHIANN
SHIANNA
SHIANNE
SHIFA
SHIFAA
SHIFAH
SHIFAN
SHIFFA
SHIFRA
SHIFRAH
SHIHAAB
SHIHAB
SHIKANA
SHIKHA
SHIKIRA
SHILA
SHILAH
SHILO
SHILOH
SHILPA
SHIMA
SHIMON
SHIN
SHINA
SHINADE
SHINAY
SHINE
SHINEAD
SHINELLE
SHINGO
SHINJI

SHION	SHLOKA	SHREY
SHIONA	SHLOME	SHREYA
SHIORI	SHLOMIE	SHREYAN
SHIR	SHLOMO	SHREYANSH
SHIRA	SHMIEL	SHREYAS
SHIRAZ	SHMUEL	SHREYASH
SHIREEN	SHNEUR	SHREYASHI
SHIREENA	SHO	SHRI
SHIREL	SHOAIB	SHRIA
SHIRELLE	SHOAN	SHRIHAN
SHIRI	SHOANA	SHRIKA
SHIRIN	SHOHAIB	SHRINA
SHIRLEY	SHOHEB	SHRIRAM
SHIRO	SHOIAB	SHRISHTI
SHIRON	SHOIB	SHRISTI
SHIRWA	SHOLA	SHRIYA
SHIV	SHOLAH	SHRIYAN
SHIVA	SHOLOM	SHRIYANS
SHIVAAN	SHOLTO	SHRUTHI
SHIVAANSH	SHOMARI	SHRUTI
SHIVAAY	SHON	SHU
SHIVALI	SHONA	SHU'AIB
SHIVAM	SHONAGH	SHUAB
SHIVAN	SHONAH	SHUAIB
SHIVANA	SHONI	SHUAYB
SHIVANGI	SHONIE	SHUBH
SHIVANI	SHONNA	SHUBHAM
SHIVANSH	SHONTAE	SHUEB
SHIVANSHI	SHONTAY	SHUGRI
SHIVANYA	SHONTELLE	SHUHAIB
SHIVAY	SHORIF	SHUHAN
SHIVEN	SHORIFA	SHUHEB
SHIVESH	SHORNA	SHUHEDA
SHIVIKA	SHOSHANA	SHUHENA
SHIVOM	SHOSHANNA	SHUJA
SHIVONNE	SHOSHONE	SHUJAAT
SHIVRAJ	SHOURYA	SHUKRI
SHIVUM	SHPETIM	SHULA
SHIYA	SHRADDHA	SHULAMIS
SHIYI	SHRAGA	SHULAMIT
SHIYING	SHRAGI	SHULEM
SHIZA	SHRAVAN	SHUMA
SHK	SHRAVYA	SHUMAILA
SHKELQIM	SHRAY	SHUMAYA
SHKO	SHRAYA	SHUME
SHLOIME	SHREE	SHUMENA
SHLOIMY	SHREENA	SHUMI
SHLOK	SHREEYA	SHUMON

SHUN	SIBELLA	SIENNA-LILY
SHURAIM	SIBGHA	SIENNA-LOUISE
SHURMA	SIBTAIN	SIENNA-MAE
SHWAN	SIBUSISO	SIENNA-MAI
SHWETA	SIBYLLA	SIENNA-MARIE
SHY	SICILY	SIENNA-MAY
SHYA	SID	SIENNA-RAE
SHYAM	SIDAL	SIENNA-ROSE
SHYAN	SIDAR	SIENNAH
SHYANE	SIDARTH	SIENNE
SHYANN	SIDDARTH	SIERA
SHYANNA	SIDDH	SIERRA
SHYANNE	SIDDHANT	SIERRA-MAE
SHYE	SIDDHANTH	SIEW
SHYHEIM	SIDDHARTH	SIGNE
SHYLA	SIDDHARTHA	SIGOURNEY
SHYLA-ROSE	SIDDHI	SIGRID
SHYLAH	SIDDIKA	SIHAAM
SHYLO	SIDDIQ	SIHAM
SHYLOH	SIDDIQA	SIHAN
SHYMA	SIDDIQAH	SIKANDAR
SHYNE	SIDDRA	SIKANDER
SHYON	SIDHARTH	SILA
SHYRA	SIDHRA	SILAN
SHYRAH	SIDI	SILAS
SI	SIDIQ	SILKA
SIA	SIDNEE	SILKE
SIAANA	SIDNEY	SILVA
SIAH	SIDNIE	SILVAN
SIAKA	SIDONA	SILVANA
SIAM	SIDONIA	SILVER
SIAMA	SIDONIE	SILVESTER
SIAN	SIDRA	SILVIA
SIAN-LOUISE	SIDRAH	SILVIE
SIAN-MARIE	SIDRATUL	SILVIO
SIANA	SIEANNA	SILVIU
SIANI	SIEGFRIED	SIMA
SIANIE	SIEM	SIMAN
SIANN	SIENA	SIMAO
SIANNA	SIENNA	SIMAR
SIANNAH	SIENNA-BEAU	SIMARAN
SIANNE	SIENNA-FAITH	SIMARDEEP
SIANTE	SIENNA-GRACE	SIMARJIT
SIARA	SIENNA-JANE	SIMARPREET
SIARAH	SIENNA-LEA	SIMAS
SIAVASH	SIENNA-LEE	SIMAY
SIBEAL	SIENNA-LEIGH	SIMBA
SIBEL	SIENNA-LILLY	SIMBARASHE

SIMBIAT
SIMCHA
SIMEON
SIMER
SIMERAN
SIMGE
SIMI
SIMILOLUWA
SIMINA
SIMISOLA
SIMMONE
SIMON
SIMONA
SIMONAS
SIMONE
SIMPHIWE
SIMRA
SIMRAH
SIMRAN
SIMRANDEEP
SIMRANJEET
SIMRANJIT
SIMRANPREET
SIMRAT
SIMRATH
SIMREET
SIMREN
SIMRIT
SIMRITA
SIMRON
SIMRUN
SIN
SINA
SINADE
SINAED
SINAI
SINAN
SINCLAIR
SINDI
SINDY
SINE
SINEAD
SINEM
SINI
SINIT
SINMILOLUWA
SINTIJA
SIOBAHN

SIOBHAIN
SIOBHAN
SIOFRA
SION
SIONA
SIONED
SIOR
SIOUXSIE
SIPHO
SIQI
SIR
SIRA
SIRAAD
SIRAAJ
SIRAC
SIRAD
SIRAH
SIRAJ
SIRAT
SIRE
SIREEN
SIRENA
SIRENNA
SIRI
SIRIN
SIRINE
SIRIOL
SIRISHA
SIRIUS
SIRUS
SISANDA
SISLEY
SISSI
SISSY
SITA
SITARA
SITI
SIU
SIUBHAN
SIVAKUMAR
SIVAN
SIVE
SIWAN
SIXTEN
SIYA
SIYAA
SIYAAM
SIYAM

SIYANA
SIYANI
SIYANNA
SIYAR
SIYARA
SIYONA
SIYU
SIYUAN
SKAISTE
SKARLET
SKARLETT
SKARLETTE
SKIE
SKY
SKY-BLUE
SKY-LOUISE
SKYANN
SKYE
SKYE-ANN
SKYE-LEIGH
SKYE-LILY
SKYE-LOUISE
SKYE-MARIE
SKYE-ROSE
SKYELA
SKYELAH
SKYIE
SKYLA
SKYLA-GRACE
SKYLA-JAE
SKYLA-JAI
SKYLA-JANE
SKYLA-LEIGH
SKYLA-LILLY
SKYLA-LOUISE
SKYLA-MAE
SKYLA-MAI
SKYLA-MARIE
SKYLA-MAY
SKYLA-RAE
SKYLA-ROSE
SKYLAH
SKYLAH-MAE
SKYLAH-RAE
SKYLAH-ROSE
SKYLAR
SKYLAR-BLUE
SKYLAR-GRACE

SKYLAR-LEIGH	SOFIA-MARIE	SOLOMIA
SKYLAR-LOUISE	SOFIA-MAY	SOLOMON
SKYLAR-MAE	SOFIA-ROSE	SOLVEIG
SKYLAR-MAI	SOFIAH	SOLYANA
SKYLAR-MARIE	SOFIAN	SOMA
SKYLAR-MAY	SOFIANE	SOMAIYA
SKYLAR-RAE	SOFIAT	SOMAN
SKYLAR-ROSE	SOFIE	SOMAYA
SKYLER	SOFIJA	SOMAYAH
SKYLER-ANN	SOFINA	SOMAYYA
SKYLER-GRACE	SOFIYA	SOMER
SKYLER-MAI	SOFIYAH	SOMERSET
SKYLER-RAE	SOFIYYA	SOMIA
SKYLER-ROSE	SOFYA	SOMKENECHUKWU
SKYLYN	SOFYAN	SOMMA
SKYRAH	SOHA	SOMMER
SKYY	SOHAAN	SOMTOCHUKWU
SLADE	SOHAIB	SOMYA
SLAINE	SOHAIL	SON
SLATER	SOHAM	SONA
SLOAN	SOHAN	SONAH
SLOANE	SOHANA	SONAKSHI
SLOKA	SOHAYB	SONAL
SMARAN	SOHEB	SONALI
SMAYAN	SOHIL	SONAM
SMILTE	SOHINI	SONAY
SMIT	SOHNA	SONDOS
SMITH	SOHRAB	SONER
SMRITI	SOHUM	SONI
SNEH	SOKAINA	SONIA
SNEHA	SOL	SONICA
SNEZANA	SOLA	SONIKA
SNIGDHA	SOLACE	SONIQUE
SNOW	SOLAL	SONITA
SOBAAN	SOLANA	SONIYA
SOBAN	SOLANGE	SONJA
SOBHAN	SOLARA	SONNA
SOBIA	SOLEIL	SONNEY
SOBIYA	SOLEN	SONNI
SOCHIMA	SOLENE	SONNIE
SOFEA	SOLENNE	SONNY
SOFFIA	SOLIANA	SONNY-JAMES
SOFI	SOLIMAN	SONNY-LEE
SOFIA	SOLIN	SONNY-RAY
SOFIA-GRACE	SOLIYANA	SONYA
SOFIA-LILLY	SOLLIE	SOOKIE
SOFIA-LOUISE	SOLLY	SOORYA
SOFIA-MAE	SOLOMAN	SOPHEA

SOPHI	SOREL	SRIKAR
SOPHIA	SOREN	SRINIDHI
SOPHIA-GRACE	SORENNA	SRINIKA
SOPHIA-JADE	SORIAH	SRINITHI
SOPHIA-LEIGH	SORIN	SRIRAM
SOPHIA-LILY	SORINA	SRISHA
SOPHIA-LOUISE	SORIYA	SRISHTI
SOPHIA-MAE	SORIYAH	SRITHARAN
SOPHIA-MAI	SOROH	SRIYA
SOPHIA-MARIE	SOROSH	SRIYAN
SOPHIA-MAY	SOROUSH	SRULI
SOPHIA-RAE	SORREL	SRULY
SOPHIA-ROSE	SORRELL	SRUTHI
SOPHIAT	SORRELLE	SRUTHY
SOPHIE	SOSAN	STACEY
SOPHIE-	SOTA	STACEY-LEIGH
SOPHIE-ANN	SOTERIS	STACI
SOPHIE-ANNE	SOTIRIA	STACIA
SOPHIE-ELLA	SOTIRIOS	STACIE
SOPHIE-ELLEN	SOTIRIS	STACY
SOPHIE-GRACE	SOUAD	STAFFORD
SOPHIE-JADE	SOUFIAN	STAISHA
SOPHIE-JANE	SOUFIANE	STAMFORD
SOPHIE-JAYNE	SOUL	STAN
SOPHIE-JO	SOULEYMANE	STAN-LEE
SOPHIE-LAUREN	SOUMAYA	STANIMIR
SOPHIE-LEA	SOUMEYA	STANISLAS
SOPHIE-LEE	SOUMIA	STANISLAV
SOPHIE-LEIGH	SOUMYA	STANISLAW
SOPHIE-LOUISE	SOURISH	STANLEE
SOPHIE-MAE	SOWMIYA	STANLEIGH
SOPHIE-MAI	SOZ	STANLEY
SOPHIE-MARIA	SPARKLE	STANLEY-JAMES
SOPHIE-MARIE	SPARSH	STANLIE
SOPHIE-MAY	SPARSHA	STANTON
SOPHIE-RAE	SPENCER	STAR
SOPHIE-ROSE	SPENSER	STARLA
SOPHIEANN	SPIKE	STARLAH
SOPHINA	SPIRIT	STARLET
SOPHIYA	SPIROS	STARLETT
SOPHY	SREE	STARR
SORA	SREENIDHI	STARZIA
SORAIA	SREEYA	STASIA
SORAIYA	SREYA	STASSY
SORAIYAH	SRI	STAVROS
SORAYA	SRIHAN	STAVROULLA
SORAYAH	SRIHARI	STEED
SORCHA	SRIJAN	STEELE

STEFAN	STEWART	SUFIYAH
STEFANI	STEWIE	SUFIYAN
STEFANIA	STILES	SUFYAAN
STEFANIE	STINA	SUFYAN
STEFANO	STIRLING	SUGA
STEFANOS	STONE	SUGHRA
STEFANY	STORM	SUGRA
STEFEN	STORME	SUHA
STEFFAN	STORY	SUHAAN
STEFFANI	STOYAN	SUHAANA
STEFFANIE	STRAWBERRY	SUHAANI
STEFFANY	STRUAN	SUHAAVI
STEFFEN	STUART	SUHAIB
STEFFI	STUTI	SUHAIL
STEISI	STYLIANOS	SUHAILA
STELA	SU	SUHAN
STELIOS	SUAAD	SUHANA
STELLA	SUAD	SUHANI
STELLAN	SUADA	SUHAS
STEPAN	SUAREZ	SUHAVI
STEPHAN	SUBAH	SUHAYB
STEPHANE	SUBAIR	SUHAYL
STEPHANI	SUBAITA	SUHAYLA
STEPHANIA	SUBAN	SUHAYLAH
STEPHANIE	SUBEER	SUHAYMA
STEPHANNIE	SUBER	SUHAYMAH
STEPHANO	SUBHA	SUHEERA
STEPHANOS	SUBHAAN	SUHEIB
STEPHANY	SUBHAN	SUHEL
STEPHEN	SUBHAN-ALI	SUHEYB
STEPHENIE	SUBHANA	SUHEYLA
STEPHY	SUBIKSHA	SUJAL
STERLING	SUBRINA	SUJAN
STEVAN	SUCCESS	SUJANA
STEVE	SUDAIS	SUJAY
STEVEN	SUDAYS	SUJITH
STEVEY	SUDE	SUJOOD
STEVI	SUDEN	SUK
STEVIE	SUDENAZ	SUKAINA
STEVIE-JO	SUDEYS	SUKAINAH
STEVIE-LEA	SUDIKSHA	SUKAYNA
STEVIE-LEE	SUE	SUKAYNAH
STEVIE-LEIGH	SUEDA	SUKEY
STEVIE-LOUISE	SUELA	SUKHBIR
STEVIE-MAE	SUFIA	SUKHDEEP
STEVIE-MAY	SUFIAN	SUKHDEV
STEVIE-RAE	SUFIYA	SUKHI
STEVIE-ROSE	SUFIYAAN	SUKHJEET

SUKHJEEVAN	SUMAIR	SUMMER-JAYNE
SUKHJINDER	SUMAIRA	SUMMER-JO
SUKHJOT	SUMAIRAA	SUMMER-LEA
SUKHLEEN	SUMAIRAH	SUMMER-LEE
SUKHMAN	SUMAIYA	SUMMER-LEIGH
SUKHMANI	SUMAIYAH	SUMMER-LILLY
SUKHPAL	SUMAIYYA	SUMMER-LILY
SUKHPREET	SUMAIYYAH	SUMMER-LOUISE
SUKHRAJ	SUMAN	SUMMER-MAE
SUKHVEER	SUMAYA	SUMMER-MAI
SUKHVINDER	SUMAYAH	SUMMER-MARIE
SUKHVIR	SUMAYIA	SUMMER-MAY
SUKHWINDER	SUMAYO	SUMMER-RAE
SUKI	SUMAYRA	SUMMER-RAY
SUKIE	SUMAYYA	SUMMER-RAYNE
SUKMANI	SUMAYYAH	SUMMER-ROSE
SUKPREET	SUMBAL	SUMMER-WILLOW
SUKRU	SUMBUL	SUMMERLEIGH
SUKVINDER	SUMEDH	SUMRAH
SULA	SUMEET	SUNA
SULAF	SUMEHRA	SUNAH
SULAIMAAN	SUMENA	SUNAINA
SULAIMAN	SUMER	SUNDAS
SULAIMON	SUMERA	SUNDAY
SULAMAN	SUMEYA	SUNDEEP
SULAYMAAN	SUMEYYE	SUNDHAS
SULAYMAN	SUMI	SUNDUS
SULDAN	SUMIA	SUNEET
SULE	SUMIT	SUNEHRA
SULEEKHA	SUMIYA	SUNETRA
SULEIMAN	SUMIYAH	SUNG
SULEKHA	SUMIYYA	SUNI
SULEMAAN	SUMIYYAH	SUNIA
SULEMAN	SUMMA	SUNIL
SULEYMAN	SUMMA-LOUISE	SUNILA
SULIAMAN	SUMMAH	SUNITA
SULIEMAN	SUMMAIYA	SUNIYA
SULIMAAN	SUMMAN	SUNJAY
SULIMAN	SUMMAR	SUNNA
SULLIVAN	SUMMAYA	SUNNAH
SULLY	SUMMAYAH	SUNNI
SULMAN	SUMMAYYAH	SUNNIE
SULTAN	SUMMER	SUNNIVA
SULTANA	SUMMER-	SUNNY
SUM	SUMMER-GRACE	SUNRAJ
SUMA	SUMMER-JADE	SUNSHINE
SUMAH	SUMMER-JANE	SUNVEER
SUMAIA	SUMMER-JAYE	SUNVIR

SUNYA
SUPRIYA
SURA
SURABHI
SURAFEL
SURAH
SURAIYA
SURAIYAH
SURAJ
SURANNE
SURAYA
SURAYAH
SURAYYA
SURAYYAH
SUREENA
SUREN
SURESH
SUREYA
SUREYYA
SURI
SURIA
SURIAH
SURINA
SURIYA
SURIYAH
SURJEET
SURRAYA
SURRAYAH
SURUTHI
SURVEEN
SURYA
SURYANSH
SUSAN
SUSANA
SUSANNA
SUSANNAH
SUSANNE
SUSHANT
SUSHMITA
SUSIE
SUTHARSAN
SUTTON
SUVAN
SUVETHA
SUVI
SUWAIBAH
SUWAYDA
SUWETHA

SUWEYDA
SUYASH
SUYEN
SUYOG
SUZAN
SUZANA
SUZANNA
SUZANNAH
SUZANNE
SUZI
SUZIE
SUZIE-MAY
SUZY
SVANA
SVANIK
SVARA
SVEA
SVEN
SVETLANA
SVETOSLAV
SVEVA
SWALEY
SWARA
SWARAN
SWARUP
SWATHI
SWATI
SWAY
SWAYAM
SWAYLEY
SWAYZE
SWETA
SWETHA
SWITHIN
SWYN
SY
SYAM
SYAN
SYANNE
SYBIL
SYBILLA
SYD
SYDELLE
SYDNEE
SYDNEY
SYDNEY-MAE
SYDNEY-RAE
SYDNEY-ROSE

SYDNI
SYDNIE
SYDONIE
SYED
SYEDA
SYEDAH
SYEDUL
SYEED
SYENNA
SYESHA
SYKE
SYLAR
SYLAS
SYLVAIN
SYLVAN
SYLVANA
SYLVESTER
SYLVI
SYLVIA
SYLVIE
SYLWESTER
SYLWIA
SYMA
SYMEON
SYMON
SYMONE
SYMPHONY
SYMRAN
SYNA
SYON
SYONA
SYRA
SYRAH
SYRENA
SYRIAH
SYRINE
SYRUS
SYYEDA
SZABOLCS
SZE
SZOFIA
SZONJA
SZYMON

T

T
T-JAY
T.
T.J.
T'JAY
T'KEYAH
T'YANNA
TA'LIYAH
TAAFEEF
TAAHA
TAAHIR
TAAHIRA
TAAIBAH
TAALIA
TAALIAH
TAALIB
TAALIYAH
TAANISH
TAANIYA
TAARA
TAARIQ
TAASEEN
TAAVI
TABAN
TABASAM
TABASOM
TABASSAM
TABASSUM
TABASUM
TABATHA
TABBITHA
TABETHA
TABINA
TABINDA
TABISH
TABITA
TABITHA
TACITA
TACY
TADAS
TADEAS
TADEUSZ
TADGH
TADHG

TADISA
TADIWA
TADIWANASHE
TAE
TAEGAN
TAEJA
TAEJAH
TAEJON
TAELA
TAELAN
TAELOR
TAEO
TAESHA
TAEVON
TAEYA
TAEYON
TAFADZWA
TAFARA
TAFARI
TAFHEEM
TAFIDA
TAHA
TAHAA
TAHAANI
TAHANI
TAHAR
TAHEED
TAHEEM
TAHEIM
TAHER
TAHERA
TAHERAH
TAHIA
TAHIBA
TAHIR
TAHIRA
TAHIRAH
TAHIRUL
TAHIRY
TAHIYA
TAHIYAH
TAHIYAT
TAHIYYA
TAHJ
TAHLA
TAHLEAH
TAHLIA
TAHLIA-ROSE

TAHLIAH
TAHLIL
TAHLIYA
TAHMEED
TAHMEENA
TAHMID
TAHMID-UR
TAHMIDA
TAHMIDUL
TAHMIDUR
TAHMIMA
TAHMIN
TAHMINA
TAHMOOR
TAHNEE
TAHREEM
TAHRIM
TAHRIMA
TAHRIN
TAHSEEN
TAHSIN
TAHSINA
TAHURA
TAHYA
TAHZEEB
TAI
TAIA
TAIAH
TAIANNE
TAIBA
TAIBAH
TAIDEN
TAIDGH
TAIF
TAIG
TAIGA
TAIGAN
TAIGEN
TAIGH
TAIJA
TAIJAH
TAIKI
TAILA
TAILAH
TAILOR
TAIM
TAIMA
TAIMOOR

TAIMUR
TAIN
TAINA
TAINE
TAIO
TAION
TAIRA
TAIS
TAISHA
TAISIA
TAISIJA
TAISIYA
TAISON
TAIT
TAITE
TAIWO
TAIYA
TAIYAB
TAIYAH
TAIYBA
TAIYO
TAIYON
TAJ
TAJA
TAJAH
TAJAUN
TAJAY
TAJINDER
TAJMINA
TAJUS
TAJVEER
TAJWAR
TAKARA
TAKIA
TAKIRA
TAKISHA
TAKIYAH
TAKONDWA
TAKSH
TAKUDZWA
TAKUDZWANASHE
TAKUMA
TAKUMI
TAKUNDA
TAKWA
TAL
TALA
TALAH
TALAHA
TALAL
TALAN
TALANA
TALAT
TALAYAH
TALAYLA
TALEA
TALEAH
TALEB
TALEEN
TALEIGHA
TALEISHA
TALEKA
TALEN
TALESHA
TALEYA
TALHA
TALHAA
TALHAH
TALI
TALIA
TALIA-LEE
TALIA-MAE
TALIA-ROSE
TALIAH
TALIAH-ROSE
TALIB
TALIESIN
TALIKA
TALIN
TALINA
TALINE
TALIS
TALISA
TALISE
TALISHA
TALISKA
TALITA
TALITHA
TALIYA
TALIYAH
TALIYAH-ROSE
TALLAN
TALLEN
TALLIA
TALLIAH
TALLIE
TALLIS
TALLIYAH
TALLON
TALLULA
TALLULAH
TALLULAH-BELLE
TALLULAH-BLU
TALLULAH-MAE
TALLULAH-RAE
TALLULAH-ROSE
TALLY
TALON
TALOR
TALULA
TALULAH
TALULLA
TALULLAH
TALVIN
TALVINDER
TALYA
TALYIA
TALYN
TALYSSA
TAM
TAMAN
TAMANA
TAMANNA
TAMANNAH
TAMAR
TAMARA
TAMARAH
TAMARI
TAMARIN
TAMARRA
TAMAS
TAMASIN
TAMAY
TAMAYA
TAMEEKA
TAMEEM
TAMEEMA
TAMEENA
TAMEIKA
TAMEIRA
TAMEKA
TAMEKAH
TAMELIA
TAMER

TAMERA
TAMESHA
TAMI
TAMIA
TAMIAH
TAMICA
TAMIE
TAMIEKA
TAMIERA
TAMIKA
TAMILA
TAMILORE
TAMIM
TAMIMA
TAMIMAH
TAMINA
TAMIR
TAMIRA
TAMIRANASHE
TAMISHA
TAMIYA
TAMIYAH
TAMJEED
TAMJID
TAMLA
TAMLIN
TAMLYN
TAMMARA
TAMMI
TAMMIE
TAMMIN
TAMMY
TAMMY-LEIGH
TAMMYLEE
TAMOOR
TAMRA
TAMRYN
TAMSEEL
TAMSIN
TAMSYN
TAMYKA
TAMZEN
TAMZID
TAMZIN
TAMZINE
TAMZYN
TAN
TANA

TANAE
TANAIYA
TANAKA
TANATSWA
TANAV
TANAY
TANAYA
TANAYAH
TANBEER
TANBIR
TANCREDI
TANE
TANEESHA
TANEISHA
TANEKA
TANEM
TANER
TANESHA
TANESHIA
TANEYA
TANGINA
TANIA
TANIAH
TANICHA
TANIELA
TANIESHA
TANIKA
TANIM
TANIMA
TANIS
TANISH
TANISHA
TANISHI
TANISHIA
TANISHKA
TANISHQ
TANISI
TANISKA
TANITA
TANITH
TANITOLUWA
TANIYA
TANIYAH
TANJA
TANJILA
TANJIM
TANJIMA
TANJINA

TANJUM
TANMAY
TANNA
TANNER
TANNIKA
TANRAJ
TANREET
TANSI
TANSIE
TANSY
TANUJ
TANUSH
TANUSHA
TANUSHKA
TANUSHRI
TANVEE
TANVEER
TANVI
TANVIKA
TANVIR
TANWEER
TANWEN
TANWIR
TANYA
TANYARADZWA
TANYEL
TANYSHA
TANZEEL
TANZEELA
TANZEELAH
TANZIA
TANZIL
TANZILA
TANZIM
TANZIMA
TANZINA
TANZY
TAO
TAOFEEK
TAOME
TAOMI
TAONA
TAONGA
TAPIWA
TAPIWANASHE
TAQI
TAQIYA
TAQIYAH

TAQWA	TARREL	TASNEEM
TAQWAA	TARRELL	TASNEEMA
TARA	TARREN	TASNEM
TARA-JADE	TARRICK	TASNIA
TARA-LEIGH	TARRIN	TASNIAH
TARA-LOUISE	TARRON	TASNIIM
TARA-MARIE	TARRYN	TASNIM
TARAH	TARUN	TASNIMA
TARAJI	TARYLL	TASNIMAH
TARAK	TARYN	TASNIYA
TARAN	TASANEE	TASNUVA
TARANA	TASARLA	TASSIA
TARANDEEP	TASEEFA	TASSNEEM
TARANEH	TASEEN	TATANIA
TARANJEET	TASFIA	TATE
TARANJIT	TASFIAH	TATENDA
TARANNUM	TASFIYAH	TATHAN
TARANPREET	TASHA	TATIANA
TARANVEER	TASHAN	TATIANNA
TARANVIR	TASHANA	TATIYANA
TARAOLUWA	TASHANI	TATJANA
TARAS	TASHANNA	TATSUYA
TAREEQ	TASHARN	TATUM
TAREK	TASHARNA	TATYANA
TARELL	TASHAUN	TATYANNA
TAREN	TASHAUNA	TAU
TAREQ	TASHFEEN	TAUFEEQ
TARIAN	TASHFIA	TAUFIQ
TARICK	TASHI	TAUHEED
TARIK	TASHIF	TAUHID
TARIKA	TASHINGA	TAUQEER
TARIN	TASHON	TAURAS
TARINA	TASHVI	TAUREN
TARINI	TASIA	TAUSEEF
TARIQ	TASKEEN	TAUSIF
TARIQUE	TASKIA	TAUTVYDAS
TARIRO	TASLEEM	TAVIA
TARJA	TASLEEMA	TAVIAN
TARKA	TASLIM	TAVION
TARKAN	TASLIMA	TAVIS
TARLIA	TASMIA	TAVISH
TARN	TASMIAH	TAVISHA
TARNYA	TASMIN	TAVLEEN
TARO	TASMINA	TAVNEET
TARON	TASMINE	TAVON
TAROOB	TASMIYA	TAVONGA
TARQUIN	TASMIYAH	TAWAB
TARRAN	TASMYN	TAWAKALITU

TAWAN
TAWANA
TAWANANYASHA
TAWANASHE
TAWANDA
TAWFEEQ
TAWFIQ
TAWHEED
TAWHID
TAWHIDA
TAWHIDUL
TAWNIE
TAWNY
TAWONGA
TAWQEER
TAWQIR
TAWSEEF
TAWSIF
TAY
TAY-YIBAH
TAYA
TAYA-LEIGH
TAYA-LOUISE
TAYA-MAE
TAYA-MAI
TAYAB
TAYABA
TAYABAH
TAYAH
TAYAH-ROSE
TAYAN
TAYANA
TAYANNA
TAYAR
TAYBA
TAYBAH
TAYDEN
TAYE
TAYEB
TAYEBA
TAYEEBA
TAYEM
TAYEN
TAYER
TAYFUN
TAYGAN
TAYHA
TAYIA
TAYIB
TAYIBA
TAYIBAH
TAYJA
TAYJAH
TAYLA
TAYLA-ANN
TAYLA-JADE
TAYLA-JO
TAYLA-LEIGH
TAYLA-MAE
TAYLA-MAI
TAYLA-MAY
TAYLA-RAE
TAYLA-ROSE
TAYLAH
TAYLAH-MAE
TAYLAH-ROSE
TAYLAN
TAYLAR
TAYLEN
TAYLER
TAYLIA
TAYLIN
TAYLON
TAYLOR
TAYLOR-
TAYLOR-ANN
TAYLOR-ANNE
TAYLOR-GRACE
TAYLOR-JACK
TAYLOR-JADE
TAYLOR-JAKE
TAYLOR-JAMES
TAYLOR-JANE
TAYLOR-JAY
TAYLOR-JAYNE
TAYLOR-JOE
TAYLOR-JOHN
TAYLOR-LEE
TAYLOR-LEIGH
TAYLOR-LOUISE
TAYLOR-MAE
TAYLOR-MAI
TAYLOR-MARIE
TAYLOR-MAY
TAYLOR-PAIGE
TAYLOR-RAE
TAYLOR-ROSE
TAYLUN
TAYM
TAYMA
TAYMAR
TAYMIYAH
TAYMIYYAH
TAYMOUR
TAYMUR
TAYNE
TAYO
TAYON
TAYSHA
TAYSHAUN
TAYSHAWN
TAYSHIA
TAYSHON
TAYSIA
TAYSIR
TAYSON
TAYT
TAYTE
TAYTEN
TAYUB
TAYVON
TAYYAB
TAYYABA
TAYYABAH
TAYYBA
TAYYBAH
TAYYEB
TAYYEBA
TAYYIB
TAYYIBA
TAYYIBAH
TAYYUB
TAZ
TAZANNA
TAZE
TAZEEM
TAZIM
TAZKIA
TAZKIYA
TAZKIYAH
TAZMEEN
TAZMIN
TAZMINE
TAZMYN

TAZNEEM	TEGWYN	TEMI
TEA	TEHANI	TEMIA
TEAGAN	TEHILA	TEMIDAYO
TEAGEN	TEHILLA	TEMIDIRE
TEAGHAN	TEHILLAH	TEMILADE
TEAGUE	TEHMEENA	TEMILAYO
TEAH	TEHMINA	TEMILOLA
TEAL	TEHMOOR	TEMILOLUWA
TEALA	TEHMUR	TEMISAN
TEALE	TEHREEM	TEMITAYO
TEAN	TEHYA	TEMITOPE
TEANA	TEHZEEB	TEMOOR
TEANNA	TEIA	TEMPANY
TEAR	TEIANA	TEMPERANCE
TED	TEIFI	TEMPERENCE
TEDD	TEIFION	TEMUJIN
TEDDI	TEIGAN	TEMUULEN
TEDDIE	TEIGE	TENAYA
TEDDIE-JAMES	TEIGEN	TENDAI
TEDDIE-LEE	TEIGHAN	TENDAYI
TEDDY	TEIGHLOR	TENDEKAI
TEDDY-JACK	TEIGUE	TENDO
TEDDY-JAMES	TEIJA	TENECIA
TEDDY-JAY	TEILA	TENESHA
TEDDY-JOHN	TEILO	TENIOLA
TEDDY-LEE	TEIRA	TENISHA
TEDDY-RAY	TEISHA	TENNESSEE
TEE	TEIYA	TENNILLE
TEE-JAY	TEJ	TENNYSON
TEEGAN	TEJA	TENULI
TEEGAN-LEIGH	TEJAH	TENZIN
TEEJAY	TEJAL	TEO
TEELA	TEJAN	TEODOR
TEESHA	TEJAS	TEODORA
TEEYA	TEJASVEER	TEODORO
TEGA	TEJASVI	TEOFILO
TEGAN	TEJASWINI	TEOMAN
TEGAN-LEIGH	TEJAY	TEON
TEGAN-LOUISE	TEJINDER	TEONA
TEGAN-MARIE	TEJPAL	TEONI
TEGBIR	TEJVEER	TEONIE
TEGEN	TEJVIR	TEQUAN
TEGH	TELERI	TEQUILA
TEGHAN	TELIA	TEQUILLA
TEGHBIR	TELISHA	TERELL
TEGHVEER	TELMO	TERELLE
TEGID	TELVIN	TERENA
TEGWEN	TEMESGEN	TERENCE

TERESA
TEREZA
TERI
TERI-ANN
TERI-ANNE
TERI-LEIGH
TERIANNE
TERINA
TERIQUE
TERRANCE
TERREL
TERRELL
TERRENCE
TERRI
TERRI-ANN
TERRI-ANNE
TERRI-LEE
TERRI-LEIGH
TERRI-LOUISE
TERRIANN
TERRIANNE
TERRIE
TERRY
TERRY-JAMES
TERRY-JUNIOR
TERTIA
TERVEL
TESHA
TESHAN
TESLIM
TESLIMAT
TESNI
TESS
TESSA
TESSIE
TESSY
TESTIMONY
TEUTA
TEVEZ
TEVIN
TEVIS
TEXAS
TEY
TEYA
TEYAH
TEYANA
TEYANNA
TEYEN
TEYHA
TEYLA
TEYMOUR
TEYONA
TEYTE
THABANI
THABISILE
THABISO
THABIT
THABO
THADDEUS
THADY
THAHERA
THAHIA
THAHIRA
THAHMINA
THAI
THAIBA
THAILA
THAINE
THAIS
THAISA
THAJ
THALEIA
THALHA
THALIA
THALIA-ROSE
THAMANNA
THAMEENA
THAMIM
THAMINA
THAMINAH
THANAA
THANBIR
THANDEKA
THANDI
THANDIE
THANDISWA
THANDIWE
THANDO
THANE
THANH
THANIA
THANISHA
THANIYA
THANJINA
THANUJAN
THANUSAN
THANUSH
THANUSHA
THANUSHAN
THANUSHKA
THANUSKA
THANVIR
THANYA
THAO
THARA
THARAN
THARANI
THARANYA
THARSHAN
THARSIGA
THARSIKA
THARUN
THARUSHI
THASHVIN
THASLIMA
THASNIM
THASWIN
THATCHER
THATO
THAYA
THE
THEA
THEA-GRACE
THEA-LOUISE
THEA-MAE
THEA-ROSE
THEADORA
THEERAN
THEERTHA
THEHAN
THEIA
THELMA
THELONIOUS
THEMBA
THENUK
THEO
THEO-GEORGE
THEO-JACK
THEO-JAMES
THEO-JOHN
THEO-LEE
THEO-PAUL
THEODEN
THEODOR

THEODORA	THOMSON	TIANA-MARIE
THEODORE	THOR	TIANA-ROSE
THEODORE-JAMES	THORA	TIANAH
THEODOROS	THORBEN	TIANE
THEOLA	THORIN	TIANEE
THEON	THORLEY	TIANEY
THEONA	THORN	TIANI
THEONI	THORNE	TIANIE
THEOPHANIA	THORNTON	TIANN
THEOPHILE	THU	TIANNA
THEOPHILUS	THULASI	TIANNA-LEIGH
THERESA	THURAYA	TIANNA-MAI
THERESE	THURAYYA	TIANNA-MARIE
THERESIA	THURSTON	TIANNA-MAY
THERON	THUY	TIANNA-ROSE
THEYA	THY	TIANNAH
THI	THYRA	TIANNE
THIA	TIA	TIANNI
THIAGO	TIA-	TIANO
THIAN	TIA-ANN	TIANYI
THIBAUD	TIA-GRACE	TIARA
THIBAULT	TIA-JADE	TIARA-LEIGH
THIBAUT	TIA-LEIGH	TIARAH
THIEN	TIA-LEONI	TIARAOLUWA
THIERNO	TIA-LOUISE	TIARN
THIERRA	TIA-MAE	TIARNA
THIERRY	TIA-MAI	TIARNA-ROSE
THIJS	TIA-MARIA	TIARNAN
THILAKSHAN	TIA-MARIE	TIARNI
THIRA	TIA-MAY	TIARNNA
THIRZA	TIA-RAE	TIARRA
THISBE	TIA-ROSE	TIAUNNA
THIVEN	TIA-SKYE	TIAYANA
THIVIYA	TIAAMII	TIBA
THIVYA	TIAAN	TIBER
THIVYAN	TIAGAN	TIBERIUS
THIYA	TIAGO	TIBOR
THOM	TIAH	TIBYAN
THOMAS	TIAHNA	TIDA
THOMAS-HENRY	TIALEIGH	TIEGAN
THOMAS-JAMES	TIAM	TIEGHAN
THOMAS-JAY	TIAMI	TIEN
THOMAS-JOHN	TIAMII	TIENNA
THOMAS-JUNIOR	TIAMO	TIERA
THOMAS-LEE	TIAN	TIERAN
THOMASIN	TIANA	TIEREN
THOMASINA	TIANA-LEIGH	TIERNAGH
THOMPSON	TIANA-MAI	TIERNAN

TIERNEY	TILLEY	TIMUR
TIERNI	TILLI	TIMURS
TIERNIE	TILLIA	TIN
TIERNY	TILLIAH	TINA
TIERON	TILLIE	TINA-MARIE
TIERRA	TILLIE-ANNE	TINARA
TIESHA	TILLIE-MAE	TINASHE
TIFANI	TILLIE-MAI	TINAYA
TIFEOLUWA	TILLIE-MAY	TINAYE
TIFFANEY	TILLIE-RAE	TINAYEISHE
TIFFANI	TILLIE-ROSE	TINESHA
TIFFANIE	TILLY	TING
TIFFANY	TILLY-	TINIKA
TIFFANY-MARIE	TILLY-ANN	TINISHA
TIFFANY-ROSE	TILLY-ANNE	TINO
TIFFINY	TILLY-GRACE	TINOTENDA
TIGAN	TILLY-JO	TIO
TIGER	TILLY-LEIGH	TIOLUWANI
TIGER-LILLY	TILLY-LOU	TIOLUWANIMI
TIGER-LILY	TILLY-LOUISE	TION
TIGER-ROSE	TILLY-MAE	TIONA
TIGERLILLY	TILLY-MAI	TIONE
TIGERLILY	TILLY-MARIE	TIONI
TIGGI	TILLY-MAY	TIONNE
TIGGY	TILLY-RAE	TIPPI
TIGHE	TILLY-ROSE	TIRA
TIHAMI	TILLY-SUE	TIRAN
TIHANA	TILLYMAE	TIRAS
TIHANNA	TILLYROSE	TIRATH
TIHOMIR	TIM	TIREE
TIIA	TIMARA	TIRENIOLUWA
TIJA	TIMAS	TIRIAN
TIJAN	TIMEA	TIRION
TIJANA	TIMEEA	TIRTH
TIJANI	TIMERA	TIRZAH
TIJEN	TIMI	TISA
TIJUS	TIMILEHIN	TISHA
TILA	TIMILEYIN	TISHAAN
TILAK	TIMMY	TISHAN
TILDA	TIMO	TISHANA
TILEAH	TIMOFEJ	TISHAUN
TILEN	TIMOFEY	TISYA
TILI	TIMON	TITAN
TILIA	TIMOTEI	TITAS
TILISA	TIMOTEJ	TITILAYO
TILISHA	TIMOTHEE	TITILOPE
TILLEE	TIMOTHY	TITO
TILLEIGH	TIMUCIN	TITOBILOLUWA

TITOBIOLUWA	TOLUNAY	TONI
TITUS	TOLUWALASE	TONI-ANN
TIVON	TOLUWALASHE	TONI-ANNE
TIWALADE	TOLUWALOPE	TONI-LEA
TIWALOLA	TOLUWANI	TONI-LEIGH
TIWALOLUWA	TOLUWANIMI	TONI-LOUISE
TIWATOPE	TOM	TONI-MARIE
TIYA	TOMA	TONI-MAY
TIYAH	TOMAS	TONIA
TIYANA	TOMASINA	TONICHA
TIYANAH	TOMASS	TONICHIA
TIYANNA	TOMASZ	TONIE
TIYARA	TOMAZ	TONIKA
TIYEN	TOMEK	TONILEE
TIZIANO	TOMER	TONILEIGH
TJ	TOMI	TONIS
TJAY	TOMI-LEE	TONISHA
TOBA	TOMIKA	TONY
TOBE	TOMISHA	TONY-JUNIOR
TOBECHI	TOMIWA	TONYA
TOBECHUKWU	TOMMAS	TOOBA
TOBENNA	TOMMASO	TOPAZ
TOBEY	TOMME	TOPRAK
TOBI	TOMMEE	TOPSY
TOBIA	TOMMI	TOR
TOBIAH	TOMMIE	TORA
TOBIAS	TOMMIE-LEE	TORAH
TOBIASZ	TOMMY	TORAL
TOBIE	TOMMY-DEAN	TORAN
TOBILOBA	TOMMY-J	TORBEN
TOBIN	TOMMY-JACK	TORE
TOBY	TOMMY-JAI	TORELL
TOBY-JAMES	TOMMY-JAMES	TOREN
TOBY-LEE	TOMMY-JAY	TOREY
TOBYN	TOMMY-JO	TORI
TOCCARA	TOMMY-JOE	TORI-LEE
TOCHI	TOMMY-JOHN	TORI-LEIGH
TOCHUKWU	TOMMY-JUNIOR	TORIA
TOD	TOMMY-LEE	TORIE
TODD	TOMMY-RAY	TORIN
TODOR	TOMMYLEE	TORITSEJU
TOHEED	TOMO	TORR
TOHURA	TOMOKA	TORRAN
TOLA	TOMOKI	TORRANCE
TOLANI	TOMOS	TORREN
TOLEEN	TOMOYA	TORRES
TOLGA	TOMS	TORRI
TOLULOPE	TONDERAI	TORRIE

TORRIN	TREYDEN	TRUPTI
TORSTEN	TREYNAE	TRYFAN
TORY	TREYON	TRYPHAENA
TORYN	TREYSON	TRYPHENA
TOSEEF	TREYVON	TRYSTAN
TOSIA	TRIANA	TSEHAY
TOULA	TRIANNA	TSELMUUN
TOURE	TRICIA	TSERING
TOUSSAINT	TRILBY	TSION
TOVA	TRIM	TSITSI
TOVE	TRINA	TSUKI
TOYA	TRINGA	TSVETAN
TOYAH	TRINITI	TUAN
TOYIN	TRINITY	TUANA
TRACEY	TRINITY-ROSE	TUBA
TRACIE	TRINNITY	TUCHE
TRACY	TRINNY	TUCKER
TRAE	TRIONA	TUDOR
TRAFFORD	TRISH	TUDUR
TRAI	TRISHA	TUESDAY
TRAN	TRISHAN	TUGBA
TRANG	TRISHANA	TUGCE
TRAVAE	TRISHNA	TUGULDUR
TRAVIS	TRISHUL	TUHEED
TRAVIS-JAMES	TRISTAN	TUI
TRAVIS-LEE	TRISTAN-JAMES	TULA
TRAVON	TRISTAN-LEE	TULAH
TRAY	TRISTEN	TULAY
TRAYVON	TRISTIAN	TULEAH
TRAYVOND	TRISTIN	TULEEN
TRE	TRISTON	TULI
TREA	TRISTRAM	TULIA
TREASURE	TRISTYN	TULIN
TREI	TRIUMPH	TULIP
TRELAWNY	TRIXIE	TULISA
TREMAINE	TROI	TULISA-MARIE
TREMAYNE	TROY	TULISA-MAY
TREMONT	TRU	TULISA-ROSE
TRENT	TRUAN	TULISE
TRENTON	TRUDI	TULISHA
TRENYCE	TRUDIE	TULISIA
TRESIAH	TRUDY	TULISSA
TREVELL	TRUE	TULLIA
TREVIN	TRULIE	TULLULAH
TREVON	TRULY	TULLY
TREVOR	TRUMAN	TULSI
TREVYN	TRUNG	TULULA
TREY	TRUONG	TULULAH

TUMELO	TYLAR	TYREEK
TUNCAY	TYLEISHA	TYREEQ
TUNDE	TYLEN	TYREES
TUNISHA	TYLER	TYREESE
TUOMAS	TYLER-	TYREISS
TUPPENCE	TYLER-DEAN	TYREKE
TURAAB	TYLER-GEORGE	TYREL
TURAN	TYLER-JACK	TYRELL
TURAYA	TYLER-JACOB	TYRELLE
TURKI	TYLER-JADE	TYREN
TURNER	TYLER-JAI	TYRESE
TUSCANY	TYLER-JAKE	TYRESSE
TUSHAR	TYLER-JAMES	TYRHYS
TUULI	TYLER-JAY	TYRIAN
TUVIA	TYLER-JOE	TYRIC
TVISHA	TYLER-JOHN	TYRICK
TWIN	TYLER-JON	TYRIECE
TWINKLE	TYLER-LEE	TYRIEK
TWISHA	TYLER-MARIE	TYRIK
TWM	TYLER-RAY	TYRIN
TWYLA	TYLER-REECE	TYRION
TY	TYLER-RHYS	TYRIQ
TY-REECE	TYLER-SCOTT	TYRIQUE
TYA	TYLERJAY	TYRON
TYAN	TYLISHA	TYRONE
TYANA	TYLO	TYRONNE
TYANNA	TYLON	TYRRELL
TYANNE	TYLOR	TYRUS
TYARNA	TYMON	TYSHA
TYBAH	TYMOTEUSZ	TYSHAUN
TYBERIUS	TYNAN	TYSON
TYCHO	TYNE	TYTUS
TYDAN	TYNESHA	TYUS
TYDE	TYNISHA	TZE
TYE	TYONA	TZIPORA
TYEE	TYR	TZIPORAH
TYEISHA	TYRA	TZIPPORA
TYELER	TYRA-LEIGH	TZIPPORAH
TYESHA	TYRAE	TZIPPY
TYGA	TYRAH	TZIREL
TYGAN	TYRAN	TZIVI
TYGER	TYREACE	TZIVIA
TYHAN	TYREAK	TZVI
TYI	TYREASE	
TYISHA	TYRECE	
TYLA	TYRECK	
TYLAH	TYREE	
TYLAN	TYREECE	

U

UBAH
UBAID
UBAIDAH
UBAIDULLAH
UBAY
UBAYD
UBAYDAH
UBAYDULLAH
UBHAY
UCHE
UCHECHI
UCHECHUKWU
UCHENNA
UDAY
UDAYSAH
UDHAM
UDIT
UDONNA
UFUK
UGBAD
UGNE
UGNIUS
UGO
UGOCHI
UGOCHUKWU
UGONNA
UGUR
UGURCAN
UISCE
UJALA
UJJWAL
ULA
ULAS
ULJANA
ULLA
ULRICH
ULRIKA
ULTAN
ULUS
ULYANA
ULYSSE
ULYSSES
UM
UMA

UMAAD
UMAAMAH
UMAAN
UMAH
UMAIMA
UMAIMAH
UMAIR
UMAIRA
UMAIRAH
UMAIS
UMAIYA
UMAIYAH
UMAIYYAH
UMAIZA
UMAMA
UMAMAH
UMANG
UMAR
UMAR-FAROOQ
UMARA
UMARAH
UMAY
UMAYA
UMAYAH
UMAYER
UMAYMA
UMAYMAH
UMAYNAH
UMAYR
UMAYRAH
UMAYYA
UMAYYAH
UMBER
UMBERTO
UME
UME-HABIBA
UMER
UMERA
UMESH
UMI
UMIKA
UMIT
UMM
UMM-E-HABIBA
UMM-E-HANI
UMMA
UMMAR
UMMAY

UMMAYAH
UMMAYYAH
UMME
UMME-HAANI
UMME-HABIBA
UMME-HABIBAH
UMME-HANI
UMMEHAANI
UMMEHANI
UMMI
UMMU
UMMUL
UMOR
UMRAH
UMRAN
UMU
UMUT
UMUTCAN
UNA
UNAI
UNAIS
UNAISA
UNAISAH
UNATHI
UNAYS
UNAYSA
UNAYSAH
UNIKA
UNIQUE
UNITY
UNNATI
UPASANA
UQBAH
URAV
URBAN
UREEBA
URENNA
URI
URIAH
URIEL
URIELLE
URIJAH
URIM
URJA
URMI
UROOJ
UROOSA
URSULA

URSZULA
URTE
URVASHI
URVI
URWA
URWAH
USAAMA
USAAMAH
USAID
USAMA
USAMAH
USAYD
USHA
USHBA
USHER
USHNA
USMA
USMAAN
USMAN
USSAMA
USWA
USWAH
UTHER
UTHMAAN
UTHMAN
UTKARSH
UTKU
UWAIS
UWAYS
UXIA
UYIOSA
UZAIR
UZAYR
UZEZI
UZMA
UZOAMAKA
UZOCHUKWU
UZOMA
UZZIAH
UZZIEL

V

VAANI
VAANIKA
VAANYA
VAARIS
VADA
VADIM
VAHID
VAHIN
VAHINI
VAIBHAV
VAIBHAVI
VAIDA
VAIDEHI
VAINAVI
VAISHALI
VAISHNAV
VAISHNAVI
VAISHVI
VAKARE
VAKARIS
VAKKAS
VALA
VALANKA
VALDEMAR
VALEN
VALENCIA
VALENTIN
VALENTINA
VALENTINA-ROSE
VALENTINE
VALENTINO
VALERIA
VALERIE
VALERIJA
VALERIO
VALERIYA
VALERY
VALI
VALMIR
VALTERS
VAMIKA
VAN
VANCE
VANDA

VANDANA
VANEESHA
VANEEZA
VANESA
VANESSA
VANI
VANIA
VANISHA
VANITA
VANSH
VANSHI
VANSHIKA
VANYA
VARANDEEP
VARIN
VARINDER
VARISHA
VARNIKA
VARSHA
VARSHAA
VARSHAN
VARSHINI
VARUN
VARVARA
VARYA
VASCO
VASIL
VASILE
VASILEIOS
VASILIA
VASILIKI
VASILIS
VASILISA
VASSILIOS
VASSOS
VAUGHAN
VAUGHN
VAYA
VAYUN
VED
VEDA
VEDAANT
VEDANSH
VEDANSHI
VEDANT
VEDANTH
VEDAT
VEDH

VEDIKA
VEENA
VEER
VEERA
VEERAJ
VEERAN
VEERPARTAP
VEGA
VEGAS
VEHAAN
VEJAS
VELA
VELI
VELIZAR
VELVET
VENA
VENBA
VENCEL
VENERA
VENESA
VENESSA
VENETIA
VENICE
VENISHA
VENITA
VENKATA
VENUS
VENYA
VERA
VERENA
VERITY
VERNON
VERON
VERONA
VERONICA
VERONIKA
VERONIQUE
VESA
VESPA
VESPER
VESTA
VESTINA
VEYA
VEYRON
VI
VIAAN
VIALLI
VIAN

VIANA
VIANNA
VIANNE
VIBHA
VIBHAV
VIBHUTI
VICENTE
VICENZO
VICKI
VICKIE
VICKY
VICTOIRE
VICTOR
VICTORIA
VICTORIA-LOUISE
VICTORINE
VICTORIOUS
VICTORY
VIDA
VIDHAN
VIDHI
VIDHUN
VIDHYA
VIDISHA
VIDUR
VIDYA
VIENNA
VIENNA-ROSE
VIERA
VIET
VIGAN
VIGGO
VIGNESH
VIGO
VIHA
VIHAAN
VIHAN
VIHANA
VIJAY
VIKAS
VIKASH
VIKASNI
VIKESH
VIKITA
VIKKI
VIKRAM
VIKRAMJIT
VIKRANT

VIKTOR
VIKTORAS
VIKTORIA
VIKTORIE
VIKTORIJA
VIKTORIYA
VIKTORS
VILIAM
VILIUS
VILLADS
VILLE
VILLO
VILTE
VIMAL
VIMBAI
VIMBAINASHE
VINA
VINAY
VINAYA
VINAYAK
VINAYKUMAR
VINCE
VINCENT
VINCENTAS
VINCENZA
VINCENZO
VINDA
VINEET
VINEETH
VINESH
VINH
VINICIUS
VINISHA
VINIT
VINITA
VINNEY
VINNI
VINNIE
VINNIE-GEORGE
VINNIE-J
VINNIE-JAY
VINNIE-LEE
VINNIE-RAY
VINNY
VINOD
VINSON
VINUDI
VINUK

VINUKI
VINUSH
VINUSHAN
VIOLA
VIOLET
VIOLET-GRACE
VIOLET-MAE
VIOLET-MAY
VIOLET-ROSE
VIOLETA
VIOLETT
VIOLETTA
VIOLETTE
VIONA
VIR
VIRA
VIRAAJ
VIRAAT
VIRAG
VIRAJ
VIRAL
VIRAN
VIRAT
VIREN
VIRGIL
VIRGINIA
VISAKAN
VISAR
VISHA
VISHAAL
VISHAKHA
VISHAL
VISHALI
VISHAN
VISHAY
VISHESH
VISHNU
VISHRUTH
VISHVA
VISHWA
VISMAY
VITA
VITALY
VITHURAN
VITHUSAN
VITHUSHA
VITHUSHAN
VITO

VITOR
VITORIA
VITTORIA
VITTORIO
VIVA
VIVAAN
VIVAN
VIVEK
VIVI
VIVIAN
VIVIANA
VIVIANE
VIVIANNA
VIVIANNE
VIVIEN
VIVIENNE
VIYA
VIYAAN
VIYAN
VIYONA
VLAD
VLADIMIR
VLADIMIRS
VLADISLAV
VLADISLAVS
VLADYSLAV
VLERA
VOGUE
VOJTECH
VOLKAN
VOLODYMYR
VOLVY
VRAJ
VRINDA
VRISHA
VRISHANK
VRISHIN
VRISHTI
VRITI
VRITIKA
VRUNDA
VRUSHTI
VSEVOLOD
VU
VUK
VUKASIN
VUONG
VUYO

VY
VYAN
VYARA
VYOM
VYTAUTAS
VYTE
VYTIS

W

WAAD
WAAIL
WAARIS
WAASIL
WADAAN
WADAN
WADE
WADI
WAEL
WAFA
WAFAA
WAFAH
WAFI
WAFIQ
WAGMA
WAHAAB
WAHAB
WAHAJ
WAHEEB
WAHEED
WAHEEDA
WAHHAJ
WAHIB
WAHIBA
WAHIBAH
WAHID
WAHIDA
WAHIDAH
WAHIDUL
WAHIDUR
WAI
WAIL
WAIN
WAIS
WAIZ
WAJAAHAT
WAJAHAT
WAJEEH
WAJEEHA
WAJID
WAJIHA
WAJIHAH
WAKAS
WALAA

WALED
WALEED
WALI
WALID
WALIULLAH
WALIYA
WALIYAH
WALKER
WALLACE
WALLIS
WALT
WALTER
WAN
WANA
WANDA
WANESSA
WANG
WANIA
WANIYA
WAQAAR
WAQAAS
WAQAR
WAQAS
WAQIA
WARD
WARDA
WARDAH
WARDAT
WAREESHA
WARICK
WARIS
WARISHA
WARISHAH
WARNAKULASURIYA
WARNER
WARREN
WARRICK
WARSAME
WARSAN
WARVAN
WARVIN
WARWICK
WASAN
WASAY
WASEEM
WASI
WASIB
WASIF

WASIL
WASIM
WASIMA
WASIQ
WASSIM
WATEEN
WAYDE
WAYLON
WAYNE
WEAAM
WEAM
WEDNESDAY
WEEAM
WEI
WEN
WENDY
WENG
WENTWORTH
WERONIKA
WESAM
WESLEY
WESMOND
WEST
WESTLEIGH
WESTLEY
WESTON
WEZLEY
WHITLEY
WHITNEY
WHITNEY-MARIE
WIAM
WICTORIA
WIDAD
WIKTOR
WIKTORIA
WIL
WILBERT
WILBUR
WILDAN
WILDER
WILEY
WILF
WILFIE
WILFRED
WILFRID
WILHELM
WILHELMINA
WILHEMINA

WILIAM
WILKIE
WILKINS
WILL
WILLA
WILLAM
WILLARD
WILLEM
WILLIAM
WILLIAM-JAMES
WILLIAMS
WILLIE
WILLIS
WILLLIAM
WILLOUGHBY
WILLOW
WILLOW-ANNE
WILLOW-FAITH
WILLOW-GRACE
WILLOW-HOPE
WILLOW-MAE
WILLOW-MAI
WILLOW-MAY
WILLOW-RAE
WILLOW-ROSE
WILLS
WILMA
WILSON
WIN
WING
WINIFRED
WINNER
WINNIE
WINNIFRED
WINNY
WINONA
WINRY
WINSLOW
WINSTON
WINTA
WINTER
WINTER-ROSE
WIOLETTA
WISAM
WISDOM
WISSAL
WISSAM
WITNEY

WITOLD
WLADYSLAW
WOJCIECH
WOJTEK
WOLF
WOLFE
WOLFGANG
WOLFIE
WOODIE
WOODROW
WOODY
WRAITH
WREN
WU
WURAOLA
WYATT
WYLIE
WYN
WYNN
WYNNE
WYNONA
WYNTER
WYNTER-ROSE
WYSTAN

X

XABI
XABIER
XAFSA
XAN
XANA
XANDA
XANDER
XANE
XANNA
XANTE
XANTHE
XANTHIA
XANTHIE
XANTIA
XARA
XARIA
XAVERY
XAVI
XAVIA
XAVIAN
XAVIAR
XAVIER
XAVIERA
XAVIERE
XAVION
XAWERY
XENA
XENIA
XENON
XERXES
XHENSILA
XHESIKA
XHOANA
XI
XIA
XIAN
XIANA
XIANG
XIAO
XIENNA
XIMENA
XIN
XING
XINYAN
XINYI
XIOMARA
XION
XSARA
XU
XUAN
XUE
XYLA
XYLIA
XYLO
XZANDER
XZAVIER

Y

YA
YA'QUB
YAA
YAACOV
YAAKOV
YAAMEEN
YAAQUB
YAARA
YAASEEN
YAASIN
YAASIR
YACIN
YACINE
YACOB
YACOOB
YACOUB
YACOV
YACQUB
YACUB
YAD
YADAV
YADAVI
YAEL
YAELLE
YAFET
YAFI
YAFIET
YAGIZ
YAGMUR
YAGO
YAHHYA
YAHIA
YAHIYA
YAHVI
YAHYA
YAHYAA
YAHYAH
YAHYE
YAIR
YAIZA
YAKIRA
YAKOB
YAKOUB
YAKOV

YAKSH
YAKUB
YAKUP
YALDA
YALIN
YALINA
YAMA
YAMAN
YAMEEN
YAMEENA
YAMEN
YAMIKANI
YAMIN
YAMINA
YAMINAH
YAMINI
YAMNA
YAMUR
YAN
YANA
YANET
YANG
YANI
YANICK
YANIK
YANIQUE
YANIS
YANKUBA
YANKY
YANN
YANNA
YANNI
YANNICK
YANNIK
YANNIS
YAO
YAPHET
YAPRAK
YAQEEN
YAQOOB
YAQOUB
YAQUB
YAQUUB
YARA
YARAH
YARAN
YARED
YAREN

YARO
YARON
YAROSLAV
YAROSLAVA
YASA
YASAMIN
YASAR
YASEEN
YASEER
YASEMIN
YASEN
YASER
YASH
YASHA
YASHAL
YASHAR
YASHAS
YASHFA
YASHFEEN
YASHI
YASHICA
YASHIKA
YASHIL
YASHITA
YASHNA
YASHNI
YASHRAJ
YASHUA
YASHVEER
YASHVI
YASHVIR
YASHWANTH
YASIIN
YASIN
YASINE
YASIR
YASIRA
YASIRAH
YASMEEN
YASMEENAH
YASMEN
YASMIN
YASMINA
YASMINE
YASMYN
YASNA
YASRA
YASSAR

YASSEEN	YESHA	YOANA
YASSER	YESHAYA	YOANN
YASSIN	YESHIKA	YOANNA
YASSINE	YESHUA	YOAV
YASSIR	YESIM	YOBEL
YASSMIN	YESSINE	YOCHANAN
YASSMINE	YESTIN	YOCHEVED
YAT	YETUNDE	YOEL
YATHARTH	YEVA	YOGESH
YAVOR	YEWANDE	YOGI
YAVUZ	YEZDA	YOHAN
YAW	YEZEN	YOHANA
YAWAR	YI	YOHANN
YAYA	YIANNA	YOHANNA
YAYRA	YIANNI	YOHANNES
YAZ	YIANNIS	YOKO
YAZAN	YICHEN	YOLANDA
YAZDAN	YIDDY	YOLANDE
YAZEED	YIDEL	YOMNA
YAZEN	YIFAN	YONA
YAZID	YIFEI	YONAEL
YAZMIN	YIGIT	YONAH
YAZMINA	YILDIZ	YONAS
YAZMINE	YILIN	YONATAN
YAZMYN	YILMAZ	YONATHAN
YE	YIN	YONG
YEA	YING	YONI
YECHESKEL	YISHAI	YONIS
YECHEZKEL	YISRAEL	YONUS
YECHIEL	YISROEL	YOONIS
YEDIDYA	YISSOCHOR	YOONSUNG
YEE	YITIAN	YOONUS
YEGOR	YITTY	YOOSUF
YEHIA	YITZCHAK	YORDAN
YEHONATAN	YITZCHOK	YORI
YEHOSHUA	YITZI	YORICK
YEHUDA	YIU	YORK
YEHUDAH	YIXIN	YOSAN
YEHUDIS	YIYANG	YOSEF
YEHYA	YIYI	YOSEPH
YEKCAN	YLANA	YOSHI
YEKTA	YLLI	YOSHUA
YELDA	YLLKA	YOSIEF
YELENA	YLVA	YOSIF
YELIZ	YNES	YOSRA
YEMAYA	YNEZ	YOSSEF
YEN	YNYR	YOSSI
YENA	YOAN	YOSUF

YOSYAS
YOTAM
YOU
YOUCEF
YOUMNA
YOUNAS
YOUNES
YOUNESS
YOUNG
YOUNIS
YOUNUS
YOURI
YOUSAF
YOUSEF
YOUSF
YOUSHA
YOUSIF
YOUSOF
YOUSRA
YOUSSEF
YOUSSOUF
YOUSUF
YOYO
YSABEAU
YSABEL
YSABELLA
YSABELLE
YSANNE
YSELLA
YSEULT
YSOBEL
YSOBELLA
YTHAN
YU
YUAN
YUBO
YUCHEN
YUDHVEER
YUE
YUEL
YUEN
YUG
YUGAN
YUGO
YUHAN
YUHAO
YUI
YUK

YUKA
YUKAI
YUKI
YUKTA
YUKTI
YUL
YULIA
YUMA
YUMI
YUMNA
YUMNAA
YUMNAH
YUN
YUNA
YUNES
YUNIS
YUNUS
YUQI
YUQIAO
YURI
YUSAF
YUSAIRAH
YUSAYRAH
YUSEF
YUSEPH
YUSHA
YUSHUA
YUSIF
YUSOF
YUSRA
YUSRAA
YUSRAH
YUSSEF
YUSSRA
YUSSUF
YUSUF
YUSUKE
YUSUPHA
YUTA
YUTIKA
YUTO
YUTONG
YUUKI
YUUSUF
YUV
YUVAAN
YUVAL
YUVAN

YUVANSH
YUVEN
YUVI
YUVIKA
YUVIN
YUVRAAJ
YUVRAJ
YUXI
YUXIN
YUXUAN
YUYA
YVA
YVAINE
YVAN
YVE
YVES
YVETTE
YVI
YVIE
YVONNE
YZABELLA

Z

Z'MARI
ZAAFIR
ZAAHID
ZAAHIR
ZAAHIRAH
ZAAKI
ZAAKIR
ZAAKIRAH
ZAAMIN
ZAARA
ZAARAH
ZAARIYA
ZABIAN
ZABIR
ZABIULLAH
ZABRINA
ZAC
ZACARIA
ZACARIAH
ZACARIAS
ZACARY
ZACCAI
ZACCARIA
ZACCARY
ZACCHAEUS
ZACH
ZACHARI
ZACHARIA
ZACHARIAH
ZACHARIAS
ZACHARIE
ZACHARIUS
ZACHARIYA
ZACHARIYAH
ZACHARY
ZACHARY-JAMES
ZACHARYA
ZACHERY
ZACHORY
ZACK
ZACKARI
ZACKARIA
ZACKARIAH
ZACKARIYA

ZACKARIYAH
ZACKARY
ZACKARYA
ZACKERY
ZADA
ZADE
ZADIE
ZADOK
ZAEEM
ZAEEMAH
ZAFAR
ZAFER
ZAFIAH
ZAFIR
ZAFIRA
ZAFIRAH
ZAFIYA
ZAFRAAN
ZAFRAN
ZAFREEN
ZAHA
ZAHAA
ZAHAN
ZAHAR
ZAHARA
ZAHED
ZAHEDA
ZAHEED
ZAHEEN
ZAHEER
ZAHEERA
ZAHER
ZAHI
ZAHIA
ZAHID
ZAHIDA
ZAHIDULLAH
ZAHIL
ZAHIN
ZAHIR
ZAHIRA
ZAHIRAH
ZAHIYA
ZAHRA
ZAHRAA
ZAHRAH
ZAHRAN
ZAI

ZAIB
ZAIB-UN-NISA
ZAIBA
ZAIBAA
ZAID
ZAIDA
ZAIDAAN
ZAIDAN
ZAIDE
ZAIDEN
ZAIGHAM
ZAIIN
ZAIL
ZAILA
ZAIM
ZAIMA
ZAIMAH
ZAIN
ZAIN-ALI
ZAIN-UL
ZAIN-UL-ABIDEEN
ZAIN-UL-ABIDIN
ZAINA
ZAINAB
ZAINAH
ZAINE
ZAINEB
ZAINIB
ZAINISH
ZAINUB
ZAINUD-DEEN
ZAINUDDIN
ZAINUDIN
ZAINUL
ZAIRA
ZAIRAH
ZAIRE
ZAISHA
ZAIYA
ZAIYAAN
ZAIYAH
ZAIYAN
ZAK
ZAKAI
ZAKAR
ZAKAREE
ZAKAREEYA
ZAKAREYA

ZAKARI
ZAKARIA
ZAKARIAH
ZAKARIAS
ZAKARIE
ZAKARIYA
ZAKARIYAH
ZAKARIYE
ZAKARIYYA
ZAKARIYYAA
ZAKARIYYAH
ZAKARY
ZAKARYA
ZAKEE
ZAKER
ZAKERIA
ZAKERIYA
ZAKERY
ZAKHARY
ZAKHIA
ZAKI
ZAKIA
ZAKIAH
ZAKIR
ZAKIRA
ZAKIRAH
ZAKIY
ZAKIYA
ZAKIYAH
ZAKIYYA
ZAKIYYAH
ZAKK
ZAKKAI
ZAKKARY
ZAKKI
ZAKKIYAH
ZAKRIA
ZAKRIYA
ZAKWAN
ZAKY
ZAL
ZALA
ZALAAN
ZALAN
ZALEKHA
ZALIKA
ZALMAN
ZALMEN
ZAM
ZAMAAN
ZAMAN
ZAMAR
ZAMEER
ZAMIL
ZAMIN
ZAMIR
ZAMIRA
ZAMZAM
ZAN
ZANA
ZANAB
ZANAIRA
ZANDA
ZANDER
ZANDILE
ZANDRA
ZANE
ZANEB
ZANELE
ZANERA
ZANETA
ZANETTA
ZANI
ZANIA
ZANIAH
ZANIB
ZANIYAH
ZANNA
ZANTHE
ZANYA
ZANYAH
ZANYAR
ZARA
ZARA-JANE
ZARA-LOUISE
ZARA-MARIA
ZARA-ROSE
ZARAAH
ZARAAN
ZARAAR
ZARAH
ZARAK
ZARAR
ZAREEN
ZAREENA
ZAREENAH
ZAREESH
ZARENA
ZARGHAM
ZARI
ZARIA
ZARIAH
ZARIF
ZARIFA
ZARIFAH
ZARIN
ZARINA
ZARINE
ZARISH
ZARIYA
ZARIYAH
ZARIYAN
ZARKA
ZARMEEN
ZAROON
ZARQA
ZARQAA
ZARRA
ZARRAH
ZARRAR
ZARRIN
ZARTASHA
ZARWA
ZARYAAB
ZARYAB
ZAVANNAH
ZAVIAN
ZAVIAR
ZAVIER
ZAVIERA
ZAVION
ZAVIYAR
ZAYA
ZAYAAN
ZAYAH
ZAYAN
ZAYANA
ZAYBA
ZAYD
ZAYDAAN
ZAYDAN
ZAYDEN
ZAYED
ZAYER

ZAYLEN	ZELAL	ZETHAN
ZAYLIE	ZELDA	ZEUS
ZAYN	ZELIA	ZEV
ZAYN-UL-ABIDIN	ZELIE	ZEVA
ZAYNA	ZELIG	ZEVI
ZAYNAB	ZELIHA	ZEYA
ZAYNAH	ZELINA	ZEYAD
ZAYNE	ZEMIRA	ZEYAN
ZAYNEB	ZEMIRAH	ZEYD
ZAYNUB	ZEN	ZEYN
ZAYON	ZENA	ZEYNA
ZAYVIER	ZENAB	ZEYNAB
ZAYYAAN	ZENAE	ZEYNAH
ZAYYAN	ZENAH	ZEYNEB
ZDENEK	ZENAT	ZEYNEP
ZE	ZENAYAH	ZHANE
ZEA	ZENDAYA	ZHANG
ZEB	ZENDEN	ZHAO
ZEBA	ZENIA	ZHARA
ZEBEDEE	ZENIB	ZHE
ZEBEDIAH	ZENITH	ZHEN
ZEBULUN	ZENIYAH	ZHENG
ZECHARIAH	ZENNA	ZHI
ZED	ZENNON	ZHIA
ZEDAN	ZENNOR	ZHIR
ZEDEKIAH	ZENO	ZHIXIN
ZEEDAN	ZENOBIA	ZHIYAN
ZEEN	ZENON	ZHONG
ZEENA	ZENTE	ZHUO
ZEENAT	ZENUB	ZHWAN
ZEENIA	ZENYA	ZHYAR
ZEESHAAN	ZEON	ZI
ZEESHAN	ZEPH	ZIA
ZEEYA	ZEPHAN	ZIAD
ZEHN	ZEPHANIAH	ZIAH
ZEHNA	ZEPHYR	ZIAN
ZEHRA	ZEPHYRUS	ZIANA
ZEIN	ZERDA	ZIANI
ZEINA	ZEREN	ZIANNA
ZEINAB	ZERIN	ZIANNE
ZEINEB	ZERINA	ZICO
ZEKAI	ZERISH	ZIDAAN
ZEKE	ZERRIN	ZIDAN
ZEKEL	ZERYA	ZIDANE
ZEKERIYA	ZESHAAN	ZIEMOWIT
ZEKI	ZESHAN	ZIENNA
ZEKIAH	ZETA	ZIGGY
ZELAH	ZETENY	ZIHAN

ZIHAO
ZIHENG
ZIKORA
ZIKRA
ZIKRAH
ZIKRIYA
ZILAN
ZILLAH
ZIMAL
ZINA
ZINAB
ZINACHIDI
ZINAR
ZINAT
ZINEB
ZINEDDINE
ZINEDINE
ZINHLE
ZINIA
ZINNEERAH
ZINNIA
ZINZILE
ZION
ZIONA
ZIPPORAH
ZIQRA
ZIRUI
ZIRWA
ZISHAAN
ZISHAN
ZISSY
ZITA
ZIVA
ZIVAH
ZIXIN
ZIXUAN
ZIYA
ZIYAAD
ZIYAAN
ZIYAD
ZIYAH
ZIYAN
ZLATA
ZLATY
ZOAIB
ZOBIA
ZOBIYA
ZOE

ZOE-ANN
ZOE-LEIGH
ZOE-LOUISE
ZOE-MARIE
ZOEY
ZOEYA
ZOFIA
ZOHA
ZOHAA
ZOHAAN
ZOHAIB
ZOHAIR
ZOHAL
ZOHAN
ZOHEB
ZOHHA
ZOHIB
ZOHRA
ZOHRAH
ZOI
ZOIE
ZOIYA
ZOJA
ZOLA
ZOLTAN
ZONA
ZONAIN
ZONAIRA
ZONERA
ZOPHIA
ZORA
ZORAH
ZORAIZ
ZORAN
ZORAVAR
ZORAWAR
ZORAYA
ZORKA
ZOSHA
ZOSIA
ZOWIE
ZOYA
ZOYAH
ZSA
ZSIGMOND
ZSOFIA
ZSOLT
ZSOMBOR

ZUBAIDA
ZUBAIDAH
ZUBAIR
ZUBAYDA
ZUBAYDAH
ZUBAYR
ZUBEDA
ZUBEIDA
ZUBEIR
ZUBER
ZUBEYDE
ZUBEYR
ZUBIA
ZUBIN
ZUHA
ZUHAA
ZUHAIB
ZUHAIR
ZUHAIRA
ZUHAIRAH
ZUHAL
ZUHAYB
ZUHAYR
ZUHAYRA
ZUHEYB
ZUHRA
ZUHUR
ZUKHRUF
ZULAIKA
ZULAIKHA
ZULAIKHAA
ZULAIKHAH
ZULAKHA
ZULAL
ZULAYKHA
ZULEIKA
ZULEIKHA
ZULEKHA
ZULEYHA
ZULFA
ZULFIKAR
ZULFIQAR
ZULKARNAIN
ZULQARNAIN
ZUMRA
ZUNAID
ZUNAIR
ZUNAIRA

ZUNAIRAH
ZUNAYRAH
ZUNDUS
ZUNERA
ZURI
ZURIEL
ZUVA
ZUWENA
ZUZA
ZUZANA
ZUZANNA
ZUZIA
ZUZU
ZVI
ZVIKOMBORERO
ZYAD
ZYAH
ZYAN
ZYANA
ZYLA
ZYLAN
ZYLUS
ZYMAL
ZYNAB
ZYNAH
ZYON
ZYRA
ZYRAH
ZYVAA